Sir Herbert Seddon

and the book he nearly didn't write

by

Julia Merrick

First published in 2010 by Fugit

British Library Cataloguing in Publication Data. A catalogue
record for this book is available from the British Library.

ISBN 978-0-9565743-0-5

The author and publisher may be contacted at:
juliamm@talktalk.net and fugit@talktalk.net

Printed and bound in the UK by Cocoa Creative Consultants

Contents

Illustrations

Acknowledgements

I am extremely grateful to Charles Macmillan junior, who had kept his father's account of a journey through England to meet Seddon, and to Churchill Livingstone, the publishers whose archives preserve the correspondence between Herbert Seddon and Charles Macmillan. Clues in those letters led me to search in libraries where I discovered more of the remarkable achievements and career of Sir Herbert. I owe thanks to Andrew Stevenson, who unintentionally started me on this venture.

In particular I am grateful to the librarians and archivists at the Royal Colleges of Surgeons in London and Edinburgh, the Churchill Archives, the Bodleian Library, the Royal Society of Medicine, the Wellcome Library, the National Library of Scotland and the Nuffield Orthopaedic Centre library.

I would also like to acknowledge the help of those who knew Seddon: David Adams, John Crawford Adams, George Bentley, Prebendary Michael Bowles, Stephanie Brooks, Robin Callendar, John Chalmers, Lord (Roger) Chorley, Max Harrison, Freddie Hicks, Ernest Jellinek, Ernest Kirwan, Alan Lettin, Ross Nicholson, Fergus Paterson, Derek Sayer and Geoffrey Walker. I apologise to the many people who worked with Herbert Seddon, but whose recollections I have not been able to include in this story.

I wish to thank those who have given permission to reproduce illustrations - especially Joan Micklem, for the portraits painted by Hugh Micklem, and Stephanie Williamson at the Institute of Orthopaedics, for photographs of the Waiting Hall at Bolsover Street. I am grateful to Andrew Stevenson at Elsevier for permission to use the correspondence from Charles Macmillan and the text and pictures from Seddon's books. Stephen Bishop at the Journal of Bone and Joint Surgery kindly gave permission to reproduce extracts from that journal. The BBC archives on line were also a valuable source. Permission was obtained from Curtis Browne to use letters from Winston Churchill. The publishers of the British Medical Journal have also been asked for permission for publication of extracts.

I would like to thank John Sisk & Sons, who kindly made a donation towards the cost of publishing. I am grateful to Herbert Seddon's children, Sally Westmacott and James Seddon, for help in many ways, to Professor Rolfe Birch for his expert comments and answers to my queries, and to Professor Kaufman for his encouragement. Gerard M-F Hill of Much Better Text expertly edited and where necessary clarified the text.

Finally, my thanks to friends and family for their comments and to my husband for his patience and photographic expertise.

Julia Merrick, May 2010

Preface

"For the Athenians and strangers which were there spent their time in nothing else, but wither to tell, or to hear some new thing" Acts 17:21

Julia Merrick has written a thoughtful and important contribution about HJ Seddon, one of the greatest clinical scientists in British Medicine. Seddon's firmness of purpose, clarity of thought, immense capacity for sustained hard work and powers of organisation were shown in "Peripheral Nerve Injuries" (1954) presented by the Nerve Injuries Committee of the Medical Research Council under his chairmanship. Both editions of Surgical Disorders of the Peripheral Nerves bear the mark of Seddon's personality: the ordered thoughts; the meticulous observation and recording; the awareness of the ambient scientific field; the occasional dogmatic assertion; the love of tabulation.

"Surgical Disorders of the Peripheral Nerves" was dedicated to the memory of two of Seddon's friends and colleagues: Hugh Cairns, Nuffield Professor of Surgery in Oxford and George Riddoch, physician to the London Hospital and the National Hospital for Nervous Diseases. In the preface to the first edition (1972) Seddon handsomely acknowledged the team of scientists with whom he worked in Oxford, including JZ Young, Peter Medawar, William Holmes, FK Sanders and Ernst Gutmann. This collaboration represents a high point in British science: from it flowed the foundation of modern concepts of the peripheral nervous system and of repair of the peripheral nerves. It was in that preface, too, that Seddon set out the qualities and the duties of the treating clinician, who should possess a wide range of skills so that the associated injuries to the skeleton, to the blood vessels, the soft tissues and the skin could be properly treated. The patient should never be in doubt about who is looking after him or her and a precise programme of treatment is all important: "Moreover, the commitment has no time limit. Ideally, the arrangement should be immune from disruption by administrative machinery". Seddon commented on the risk of rejecting established proven and reliable techniques in favour of what is novel and he argued for the controlled clinical trial, "one of the most weighty weapons of contemporary research". Indeed Seddon was the driving force for the trial of different methods of treatment of tuberculosis of the spine, under the auspices of the Medical Research Committee, a project extending over ten years of work and which involved many workers.

The intellectual and clinical strengths which were such a remarkable characteristic of Seddon's work had their effect on the many young men and women who worked with him and who were trained by him. Many went on to make substantial contributions in different branches of medicine. In latter years his tenure at the Royal National Orthopaedic Hospital undoubtedly represented an apogee for that Institution as it was for British orthopaedics.

The biography written by Julia Merrick draws on much hitherto unpublished material and correspondence with those who knew him and those who worked with him. The extensive correspondence with his publishers, Churchill Livingstone, suggests, at first sight, the courtesy of a bygone age but they also reflect a consistent commitment by those involved which still stands as an example.

Rolfe Birch
Stanmore

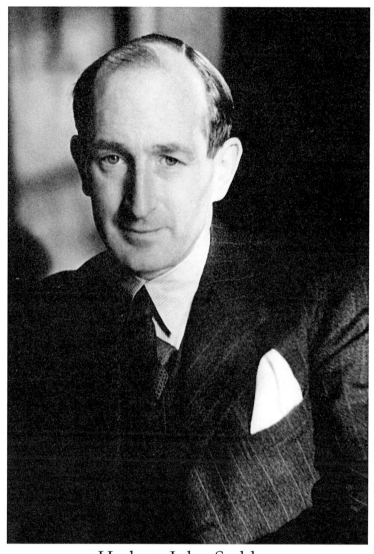

Herbert John Seddon

Introduction

This is the story of an outstanding surgeon, Sir Herbert Seddon (1903-1977), a pioneer in two fields of surgery: the understanding and treatment of crippling diseases, notably tuberculosis and poliomyelitis, where many of his patients were children, and the repair of severe injury to peripheral nerves. In both fields he learnt rapidly because cases were so numerous at the time.

Seddon's first success, as a young surgeon at the Royal National Orthopaedic Hospital, was in understanding spinal deformities caused by the tuberculosis bacillus, and this led to progress in surgical treatment. He applied scientific logic to the damage caused by disease, but he also gained a reputation for his empathy with and intelligent response to his many young patients.

At the age of only 36, he was appointed to a chair at Oxford, where he worked alongside leading scientists. It was 1940, and he was appointed specifically to establish a peripheral nerve injury unit, so almost at once he had to deal with the casualties of war. This gave Herbert Seddon the chance to become a master at repairing injury to peripheral nerves. He would have known that there was a history of of thousands of years of surgeons perfecting their skills as a result of war. During wartime epidemics of polio he was sent to the colonies to advise on policy and treatment. Post-war, his authority and ambitions at Oxford were questioned. He considered his position at the Wingfield-Morris Hospital had become untenable, but fortunately he was able to return to the Royal National Orthopaedic Hospital and the Institute of Orthopaedics as Director. He was instrumental in developing specialist fields of orthopaedic surgery and made the hospital internationally renowned, welcoming visitors from around the world and exporting highly qualified orthopaedic surgeons. He worked hard, influenced a generation of young surgeons, travelled widely and treated interesting patients, both from a clinical point and from their character or celebrity.

This is also the story of a book, Seddon's *magnum opus*, and its thirty-year gestation. He published far more than the average surgeon of the time, but his early enthusiasm to write a book on the disorders of peripheral nerves was continually delayed by his successful surgical and academic career, despite frequent encouragement from the publisher Charles Macmillan. Only when he retired was the book completed and published in 1972 to widespread acclaim.

That I uncovered the history of Herbert Seddon at all is thanks to Charles Macmillan, who kept a record of all their correspondence. I found these letters in the archives of Churchill Livingstone, yet they contain no other correspondence between an author and the publisher. Charles Macmillan must have valued his friendship with Seddon quite as much as the book that finally resulted from his persistent encouragement.

Macmillan played a significant part in publicising the work of surgeons. He was just one year older than Seddon, a likeable and enthusiastic man who often saw the amusing side of events. After working for the printers Thomas Nelson & Sons, in 1919 he joined E & S Livingstone, medical publishers and booksellers, at their office opposite the University of Edinburgh Medical School. He married in 1930 and started a family. In 1937 he was appointed general manager of E & S Livingstone. Charles Macmillan junior kept his father's report of the publisher's journey in 1941 to meet Seddon.

Like a tailor, the publisher must present the surgeon to the world in the best possible way. The surgeon's work must be explained in detail, the information must be clearly represented, the book must be fit for purpose and affordable. The publisher has to coax and encourage the author, be sympathetic to his problems and persuade him to delegate responsibility so he can concentrate on writing. The publisher must also help the surgeon to choose the moment to complete the book, the moment when he has reached a peak of knowledge and expertise, so that his book will become a classic in its field. The publisher may defer to the brilliant surgeon, but the publisher's judgement and skill – editorial, production and marketing – play an important part in the dissemination of medical knowledge.

In this case the surgeon and publisher got to know each other well over the course of thirty years. The result of the partnership between Seddon and Macmillan is one of the great classics of surgery and today a rare book in its original form. The title is still in print, though the content has been updated and rewritten.

Chapter 1

How Herbert Seddon became an orthopaedic surgeon

Herbert John Seddon was born on 13 July 1903, the first son of John Seddon, sales manager for Union Cold Storage in London, and Ellen *née* Thornton. His parents moved to the north of England, first to Derby and then to Manchester. After being turned down by Manchester Grammar School, he was educated at Hulme Grammar School, where he decided to choose medicine as a career.

He went on to study medicine at Barts – St Bartholomew's Hospital and Medical School, London – and obtained MB, BS. He already showed promise of a great future, winning a fistful of scholarships: in Anatomy and Physiology, the Harvey Prize for Practical Physiology, the Brackenbury Scholarship in General Surgery, the Foster Prize for Anatomical Dissection, the Walshar Prize for Surgical Pathology and the Willmot Medal for Operative Surgery. In 1928 he was awarded the London University Gold Medal.[1] Aged only 23 he had a case published in the British Journal of Surgery with GL Alexander as first author.[2]

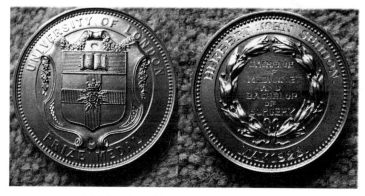

1. University of London Gold Medal 1928

1 University of Oxford Archives UR6/MD/13/8.
2 Alexander GL and Seddon HJ 1926.

He decided on a career in surgery and took the examinations to become a fellow of the Royal College of Surgeons of England (FRCS). Seddon's mentor at Barts had been Reginald Cheyne Elmslie, who took a particularly scientific approach to orthopaedics, emphasising the need to understand the pathology causing the diseases that the surgeon treated. For Seddon, whose first love had been chemistry, this approach was most welcome. Other students of Elmslie to achieve prominence in orthopaedics were Capener, Higgs and Jackson Burrows and all three would work with or at least exchange important ideas with Seddon.

As a young orthopaedic surgeon Seddon joined the British Orthopaedic Association where he met Sir Robert Jones, a great pioneer of orthopaedic surgery. Seddon described the occasion:

> My first appearance at the British Orthopaedic Association was his last. I remember it clearly. There he sat in patriarchal splendour, surrounded by his favourite sons, Bristow, Girdlestone, McMurray, Platt and Malkin, to name only a few among them. In those days the Association was a small affair, something of a club; its spontaneity was not blighted by a microphone. We youngsters in the back row noted every word, the astonishing wisdom of Sir Robert's remarks, the geniality that softened the blow of a devastating question.
>
> Later we gathered round him – the attraction was quite irresistible – and he asked us about our work with an interest and understanding too genuine, too friendly to be mere flattering. We felt that we were the grandchildren.[3]

In 1928 Seddon was appointed to a registrar post at the Royal National Orthopaedic Hospital at Stanmore. The hospital was on Brockley Hill, north-west of London (now just inside the M25) and only a short train journey away from town and the Great Portland Street branch of the hospital. An additional attraction was the Royal Society of Medicine, a club with an excellent library. There he was able to attend meetings of the Orthopaedic Section; he became a member of the section in April 1929, at the same time as

---

3 Seddon 1961b.

William Muir Dickson. There were just three or four meetings a year, held in the evening at the club in Wimpole Street. Interesting cases were demonstrated and discussed.

Surgery is a craft best learnt by watching a master operate, and the keen novice has traditionally travelled to find experts to observe. At this time many young doctors were attracted to North America, so much so that a recognised milestone in their careers was gaining what came to be known as BTA or 'Been to America'. So, after a short time in Stanmore, Seddon obtained a post as Instructor in Surgery at Ann Arbor, Michigan, where Carl Badgley was the orthopaedic surgeon and inspirational teacher.[4] Seddon asked for permission to go there in 1930, was granted leave and told he could return as a registrar in the London part of the RNOH in Great Portland Street. While in America he visited many of the leading professionals: Dr Steindler in Iowa City, Mr Henderson in the Mayo Clinic, Professor Gallie in Toronto and Dr Russell Hibbi in New York. He also went to the Massachusetts General Hospital in Boston, to see how fractures were treated there, and to the children's hospital.[5]

At Ann Arbor he was attracted to a house mother of students, Mary Lorene Lytle, who came from from Marquette in Michigan. Not wanting to call him Herbert, a name he disliked, she asked what the J stood for. He would not tell, she guessed James and so called him Jim, a name that stuck among friends and family. They married and a daughter named Sally was born in 1935 and nearly three years later a son called James. An ophthalmologist and Olympic athlete Hyla Stallard, known as Henry, who was a friend from Seddon's student days at Barts, was invited to be godfather to James.

Of slight build and average height, Seddon was neither conventionally handsome, nor the flamboyant theatrical figure of the fictional surgeon. He had blue eyes and a nose that was rather too long and narrow, and dark hair which soon thinned and turned grey. His interests were many. He joined the Fell and Rock Climbing Club, a Lake District group. Before and during the war he climbed in Wasdale with one of his neighbours who lived at the top of Stanmore Hill, Lord Chorley. His son Roger caught polio, but made a good recovery. It must have been reassuring to have advice from a

---

4 S, 'Obituary: Carl Badgley', *JBJS*, **55A** (1973) 5.
5 University of Oxford Archives, UR6/MD/13/8.

friend like 'Jim'. Another of Seddon's climbing friends was AM Binnie, a don at the engineering department in the University of Cambridge who later taught James when he was a student there. Seddon enjoyed the exotic landscapes he saw on foreign visits, took photographs and later in his life used them as subjects for painting. He also made his own black-and-white photographic prints. Seddon appreciated music and played bridge with family and friends. Among the neighbours at Stanmore whom he came to know was Clement Attlee. He admired this politician and post-war prime minister for his determination to better the conditions of the working class.

In 1931 the hospital at Stanmore had 320 beds, half of them for surgical tuberculosis cases, and it was expanding. Soon after Seddon returned to England, he was invited to fill the vacant post of Resident Surgeon and Medical Superintendent there. In those days consultants visited their patients only about once a fortnight so the main responsibility for care rested with him. Elmslie, for whom he had worked, had recommended that the Committee of Management select Seddon. The patronage of a senior member of the profession was important for a young surgeon and, when compounded with ability, gave a sure indication of a successful future. Seddon invited John Cholmeley, another Barts graduate, to apply for the post of assistant resident surgeon.

At the beginning of April 1935 his keenness was recognised and he was nominated to the Council of the Orthopaedic Section of the Royal Society of Medicine (RSM). For the next two years he regularly attended the council meetings and was elected the Honorary Secretary – an office he shared with Norman Capener. He was then appointed Library Representative to replace Laming Evans, who was "going abroad for a time" (about a year).

Observation, classification and method of treatment were the three steps in the scientific approach to disease, and there was plenty of material for the dedicated young orthopaedic surgeon to work on and publish.[6] Eponyms had been given to some combinations of abnormalities, and the true significance of these could be re-examined. At the meetings, open to all members of the RSM and held at Wimpole Street on Tuesdays at 5.30 p.m., Seddon and his colleagues demonstrated a variety of cases to an audience of about a

6 Seddon 1930, 1932a, 1934, 1935b.

hundred people.[7]

> 5 November 1935: three cases shown by Seddon
> Report on fatal case of empyema secondary to a
> tuberculous spinal abscess
> Report on a case of rupture of a tuberculous spinal
> abscess into the oesophagus
> Osteochondritis of the base of the first metatarsal bone
> 6 October 1936: Seddon showed two cases of the eight
> presented that evening
> Traumatic brachial paralysis
> Multiple neuro-fibromata with deposits in long bones and
> scoliosis [also known as Von Recklinghausen's disease]
> 3 November 1936: Seddon showed one case of four
> Aseptic necrosis of the femoral head of a child
> 5 January 1937: Seddon showed one case of ten
> Slipped femoral epiphysis
> 4 May 1937: Seddon showed one of eight cases
> Spondylolisthesis in a girl of 15 years
> 5 October 1937: Seddon showed one of nine cases
> Specimen from a case of Pott's paraplegia
> 2 May 1939: Seddon showed cases of diffuse neuroma of the
> arm and extensive ulceration of arm.
> (His report of this case was submitted to Nature).

More work was published.[8] This part of Seddon's career was the foundation for later work,[9] as Professor JIP James recalls in his obituary:

> It was while at Stanmore that he made his initial con-
> tribution to the pathology of paraplegia in spinal tuber-
> culosis. He clarified the pathogenesis of paraplegia and
> showed clearly that it was due to the intervertebral
> abscess bulging backwards against the cord, and that it
> was not the kyphosis that caused cord damage. He also
> distinguished between this early, acute paraplegia due

---

7 RSM archives of the Orthopaedic Section.
8 Seddon 1936a, 1937, 1938a, 1938b, 1939.
9 Seddon 1946b, Griffiths, Seddon and Roaf 1956.

to an abscess and late onset paraplegia due to gliosis secondary to a long-standing kyphosis and ischaemia[10]

Percival Pott, an eighteenth-century Barts surgeon, had described the damage to the spine;[11] now Seddon had explained the causes. In 1938 the Council of the Chartered Society of Massage and Medical Gymnastics co-opted the help of Seddon and he became Honorary Secretary of the orthopaedics section of the British Medical Association (BMA).

In 1939 Mary, Jim and the two children were in America with her parents. Their wooden house overlooking Lake Superior was a beautiful and peaceful refuge. Seddon took the opportunity to do some work at a hospital in Marquette, but returned to England alone when war was declared. There the need to provide services for war-wounded patients led Seddon into a different area of orthopaedics: the repair of peripheral nerves. Following the outbreak of war, the Council of the RSM decided on 3 October 1939 to continue to hold meetings of the section "as long as conditions would permit". It was 'conditions' like aerial bombardment or even invasion that many people feared, so at the start of the war many children were evacuated from London to the country, only to return a few weeks later.

The term 'orthopaedic' derives from the Greek words for 'right or straight' and 'child', and in the early days the work of the orthopaedic surgeon had been to address child deformities, commonly caused by rickets. The work extended to treating paralysis of fingers, arms and legs. So it was that, when war wounds required the repair of peripheral nerves, the general surgeon needed the skills of the orthopaedic specialist. This is just one example of how the career of the general surgeon in the twentieth century was carved up and served as a delicacy to specialist surgeons: ears, noses and throats, kidneys, reproductive systems, livers and hearts all acquired specialist surgeons who would discover new methods and as chiefs – or 'chefs' – would teach the next generation of surgeons. Peripheral nerve surgery remained a dish for the orthopaedic surgeon for the next half century.

The treatment of nerve injuries had been under the care of orthopaedic surgeons since the First World War. Treatment centres

---

10 James 1978.
11 Pott 1779.

had been set up by Sir Robert Jones at Alder Hey in Liverpool and at Shepherds Bush in London, but after that war it was impossible to follow up the results of those cases, and records were inadequate for future research. In 1923 Harry Platt and Rowley Bristow concluded that only the joining of nerves end to end had any marked success; grafts to fill gaps had been a failure. Moreover, Bristow was not optimistic about future progress.[12] Now, for the Second World War, a Nerve Injuries Committee of the Medical Research Council was convened to address these problems. George Riddoch, a neurologist, was in the chair and he was determined that this time cases would be thoroughly recorded. Also, with the help of the Ministry of Pensions, follow-up was to be continued for several years (in fact until 1949).[13] George Riddoch had experience of running a hospital in the First World War and afterwards he worked at the London Hospital where he became head of the neurology unit.

It was understood, when war seemed likely, that specialist units for peripheral nerve injuries would be needed across the country. Five hospitals were made centres for treatment: Botley Park Emergency Hospital in Chertsey was headed by Brigadier WR Bristow; Winwick Emergency Hospital in Warrington had Professor Sir Harry Platt as chief surgeon; Seddon was invited to be head of the third, in Oxford; in Scotland the Emergency Medical Services (EMS) Hospital at Killean near Glasgow had CRW Illingworth and fifthly the EMS Hospital at Gogarburn near Edinburgh had Professor Learmonth. He and Bristow were of the older generation of orthopaedic surgeons who had served in the First World War. The two Scottish centres were not part of an orthopaedic hospital.

Other catalysts of Seddon's move to Oxford were at work. Lord Nuffield, or William Morris as he had been known, had made a fortune from making cars in Oxford. Before the war he had been a most generous benefactor to medicine. He had purchased for the university the elegant old observatory building next to the Radcliffe Infirmary, to be used for clinical research. In war, at the request of Brigadier Cairns RAMC, he was having mobile surgical units constructed for the Royal Canadian Army Medical Corps in 3 ton motor vehicles with four-wheel drive and electric generators.

Nuffield funded a number of chairs in Oxford, and Hugh

---

12 Platt and Bristow 1923.
13 Seddon and Riddoch 1953.

Cairns had been selected as the first Nuffield Professor of Surgery in 1937. As well as studying in England (he was Australian by birth) he had spent some time learning the methods of Harvey Cushing in Boston and he was keen to establish neurosurgery as a separate specialty. Colonel (later Brigadier) Cairns excelled as an organiser of immense energy and was appointed Consultant for Neurological Services to the Director General of Medical Services of the British Army. In this capacity he designed and administered mobile neurosurgical units to treat casualties near the front line and established a Combined Services Hospital for Head Injuries in the relatively modern building of the women's college St Hugh's.[14] The injured were flown to Brize Norton and then had a relatively short onward journey to Oxford. There was also an airport for Oxford at Kidlington, opened in 1938.

Far from being the famed 'city of dreaming spires', at this time Oxford was more like a volcano: some areas were asleep, but others were turbulent, not only producing brilliant eruptions of new discoveries but also smouldering with rivalries. Its physical shape was changing too, as people flowed like lava into requisitioned college buildings and temporary hutted accommodation, while others left to join the armed services.

The locally well-known and loved benefactor and surgeon Gathorne Robert Girdlestone stepped down from the Nuffield-funded chair in orthopaedics, to make room for a younger man who would also be the Clinical Director at the Wingfield-Morris Hospital but Girdlestone would continue as an honorary surgeon there. The hospital was quite modern since the original collection of wooden huts had been replaced by light and airy brick pavilions, declared open by the Prince of Wales in 1933. Patients were admitted from several nearby counties as well as Oxfordshire. In the terminology of the day they included 'crippled' children, people with non-pulmonary tuberculosis or 'infantile paralysis' (poliomyelitis), and patients with severe injuries of the spine and limbs. The hospital had its own work-shops to supply appliances to the surgeons' order and 'crippled' young men were given training there. War wounded were brought to the hospital for specialist treatment. There was a separate ward 'Nani' for the officers and a ward of about ten beds for private patients,

---

14 Davis 1964.

nicknamed Mayfair. Compound fractures of the extremities and severe burns were treated at the Radcliffe Infirmary. An annexe for an extra 70 patients was opened at Ripon Hall on the edge of Oxford.

Seddon's ability was recognised by Professor Girdlestone, who invited him to apply for the post of professor that Girdlestone had vacated. Other applicants were considered, but Seddon was appointed as Nuffield Professor of Orthopaedics and a professorial fellow of Worcester College, Oxford. He took up his post in January 1940 with the necessary matriculation at the university on 30 January. That day he was awarded MA and DM, both by decree. In February he was made a member of the Nuffield Committee for the Advancement of Medicine. Seddon's abilities had led him to positions of power and influence, but his future path was not so straightforward.

The peripheral nerve injury unit was a sub-specialty of orthopaedics and not of neurosurgery, but the two professors, Seddon and Brigadier Cairns, had frequent contact. Seddon learnt from Cairns "a delicacy of touch that lies between those of the neurosurgeon and the otologist" and from George Riddoch "the special skills – and patience – of the neurologist".[15] "Wee Georgie" was an Aberdonian graduate with a dry sense of humour and plenty of energy until his later years, when he became sadly debilitated by a gastric ulcer. He died post-operatively in 1947.

At the same time as Seddon was setting up his unit at the Wingfield-Morris, other hospitals were being organised to treat the war wounded and buildings were being requisitioned to house convalescent patients. Near the Wingfield-Morris Hospital, the new Churchill Hospital was under construction. The Warneford and Park hospitals for the mentally ill were also in Headington. Oxford was a busy medical centre with the Radcliffe Infirmary, the teaching hospital, at the centre of the city. In hospitals and in the university new methods of treatment were being explored.

Lord and Lady Bicester offered hospitality in Oxford to Seddon when he first arrived. Their daughter Dr the Honourable Honor Smith was a physician specialising in tubercular meningitis with whom Seddon collaborated. He soon found an ideal house

---

15 Preface in Seddon 1972.

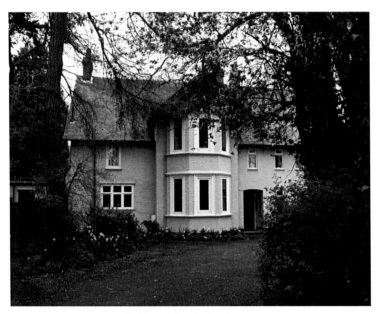

2. 66 Old Road Headington

opposite the Wingfield-Morris Hospital in Headington. At £2,000, it cost little more than a year's salary. His parents moved to Oxford to live with him while Mary and the children were still in America. His Lancashire father died after a short time in Oxford, but his Yorkshire mother, Ellen (*née* Thornton) lived to play an important role as hostess for him. She cooked a great traditional Sunday dinner of roast beef and Yorkshire pudding, sometimes serving the latter as a dessert with golden syrup. She would delight in teasing her son "the Professor" but was really so proud of him. On weekdays she would send their maid round to the hospital with some home-made cakes or scones for his tea.

Some evenings he dined in the elegant hall of Worcester College and socialised with the other fellows – all from the arts faculties – whose company was a welcome escape from the pressure of work. The crisp, elegant eighteenth-century façade of the college in Beaumont Street, built in a soft golden stone, was crumbling. Lord Nuffield preferred to put money into a brand-new building and

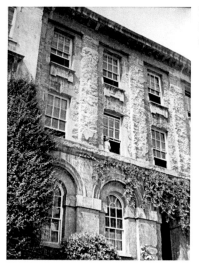

3. Crumbling stones at Worcester College (detail of S. front), Oxford, in the 1930s

medical scholarships, not into restoration. The Oxford colleges kept excellent cellars and Seddon learnt to appreciate fine wines, an enthusiasm he followed up in later years on visits to France, even becoming a *chevalier du vin*. It was probably at this time that he became a member of the Athenaeum Club in London.

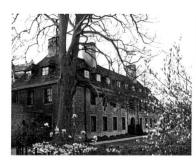
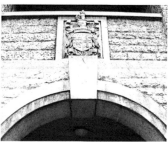

4. Nuffield Institute at Worcester College

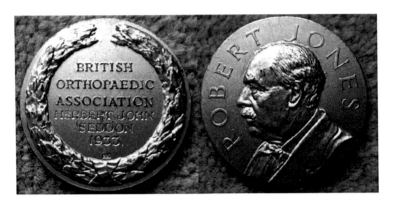

5. Robert Jones Medal

In 1940 Charles Macmillan of E & S Livingstone was casting around for new authors who could write about the treatment of war injuries. One possible candidate, who had approached him with an idea for a book, was that new Nuffield Professor of Orthopaedics in Oxford. In considering whether Herbert Seddon would be an able author, Charles Macmillan only had to look at the Robert Jones Prize Essay on 'Pott's Paraplegia' by Seddon (1934), preceded by one by R Weedon Butler, Honorary Surgeon at Addenbrookes Hospital, Cambridge, with whom he shared the prize, or to read Seddon's 'Morbid anatomy of caries of the thoracic spine in relation to treatment' published in *The Lancet* (1935).

The latter had been first given as the Hunterian Lecture at the Royal College of Surgeons of England, a most prestigious invitation. The research was thorough, the prose was lucid, an anatomically inaccurate term 'epiphyseal tuberculosis' was rejected in favour of 'metaphysis tuberculosis' and the drawings were clear, though Macmillan may have blanched at the photograph of the Stanmore frame, on which a figure is held spine arched backwards in traction, or the "plaster shell, carrying post for attachment of skull-traction appliance". Less frightening was a device made with rubber tubes and detachable posts "to prevent foot-drop while preserving a range of movement". This was the realm of orthopaedics. The quality of the X-ray pictures was also good and acknowledged by Seddon.

Macmillan appreciated the sales value of good illustration in his company's text books. He began discussion with Professor Seddon on the publication of a book about the treatment of peripheral nerve injuries.

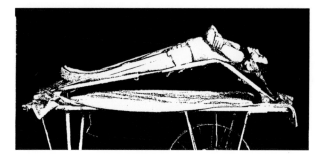

6. The Stanmore Frame

Chapter 2

Charles Macmillan visits his authors and signs Seddon

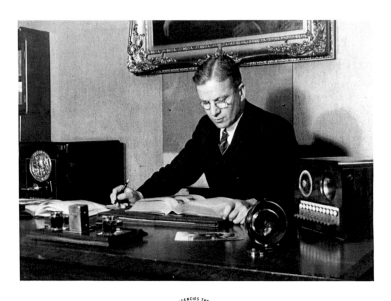

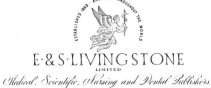

7. Charles Macmillan at his desk and
E & S Livingstone letterhead

CM/NMB   24th September, 1941.

Dear Professor Seddon,
    As promised, I have pleasure in writing to inform you that my firm will be delighted to publish your new book dealing with Peripheral Nerve Injuries.
    I therefore trust that you will make steady progress in its compilation, and as soon as you require any assistance from me, I trust you will not hesitate to communicate with me.....
    I have pleasure in sending you two documents which were prepared for Professor Illingworth's "Textbook of Surgical Treatment".[16] The first note was sent to the contributors giving them a general idea of the scope of the book and the editorial arrangements.
    After they had agreed to take part, then the detailed contents were arranged, and a certain number of words allocated to each chapter and also the number of illustrations clearly stated. This was sent to the contributor at a later date to make sure that there would be no such thing as overlapping.
    Although I am certain that this original detailed contents was not strictly adhered to, it served as a means of guidance for each contributor.
    If you could draw up similar documents which could be used for the British Textbook of Orthopaedics and submit these to Professor Platt and at the same time inform him of Mr Watson-Jones' intention of writing a companion book to his Fractures, on Orthopaedic Surgery as soon as an opportunity presented itself, this might stir Professor Platt into action.[17]
    As I stated, I do not think Mr. Watson-Jones will have the time or opportunity during war time to go forward with this new venture. If this book was arranged and some progress made with it, it would certainly damp his enthusiasm. I therefore leave this matter with you and I shall be interested to hear of any future developments.
    I would take this opportunity of thanking you for the courtesy you showed me at my interview, and it is

16 Charles Illingworth, Regius Professor of Surgery in the University of Glasgow, treated peripheral nerve injuries there.

extremely kind of you to pay such high tribute to our
firm in producing beautiful medical Textbooks.
    I am,
           Yours sincerely,
               for E. & S. Livingstone,
                  Charles Macmillan
                     Manager.
Professor H.J. Seddon, F.R.C.S.,
Brockley House, Old Road,
    Headington, Oxford.

Macmillan wrote this letter the day after coming back from
a week of travel through England and Wales visiting surgical and
medical authors, bookshops and a government office. The report he
wrote for his firm was much more than the talk of contributors,
payments, chapters and headings that one might expect. It is a
publisher's tour of leading surgeons of the day, whose fame was
known by Seddon, and an adventure through war-damaged England
that vividly portrays the way of life and the state of the country at
that time. With Macmillan as guide, we can plunge back into the
idioms of another time and, like Alice in Wonderland, discover some
eccentricities.

---

17   Reginald Watson-Jones, a contemporary of Seddon in
Liverpool, was one of the first surgeons to take the specialist degree
M.Ch.Orth. Robert Jones saw his potential. As Civilian Consultant in
Orthopaedic Surgery to the RAF, Watson-Jones helped set up a network
of orthopaedic units in Britain and abroad, combining these with four
major rehabilitation units that got many men with injured ligaments
back into service. On top of his extensive private practice, lecturing and
writing, he served on the MRC war wounds committee. Despite needing
little sleep, he was fully stretched at this time. Watson-Jones worked
closely with Harry Platt in Manchester. They replaced scribbled medical
notes with legible typed ones. Harry Platt, a generation older, was a
major figure who had been president of the British Orthopaedic
Association in 1934. He was founding editor of the *Journal of Bone and
Joint Surgery* and assistant consultant adviser in orthopaedic surgery to
the Ministry of Health. He played an important part in establishing the
American Hospital, which moved to the Churchill Hospital in 1942.

CM/NMB
25.9.41
PARTICULARS OF MY VISIT DOWN SOUTH.
<u>Friday 12th to Saturday 20th September.</u>
I left Princes Street Station with the 10.55 train, which left promptly and was not over-crowded. At Carlisle, however, the train was comfortably filled. At Aintree we had to change trains, and an electric train took us right into Exchange Station.

As we passed through Bootle and Kirkdale, I saw how colossal was the damage to property, factories and warehouses, I have never seen anything that made me feel so sad. Hundreds of beautiful homes are simply laid flat, great big factories – only the shells of buildings left. On making enquiries at Liverpool, I found that there are still over 4,000 families homeless. The week of continuous air raids resulted in 3,000 people being certified dead at the various hospitals, and this did not include the number of persons who were buried alive. Liverpool is in a very bad way indeed.

Dr Coope met Macmillan and drove him in an old Rolls-Royce to his country cottage in Eales to discuss a book on 'Diseases of the Chest'. From there, Macmillan continued by train:

I travelled back from Wales to a junction called Hooton. From there I took the train to Birkenhead, crossed the Mersey on one of the ferry boats, saw a large convoy coming in from America, and observed large cases which I felt contained aeroplanes, set right along the roads, about 50 yards apart. I think the idea was that there would be less chance of them all being damaged in the event of a blitz. The convoy consisted of about 50 ships and there was extreme activity round about the docks.

After a quiet weekend with friends, Macmillan was back to work in Liverpool tracking down possible authors:

First thing on Monday morning, I was busy trying to make appointments. After four telephone calls, I managed to arrange to see Dr. Thompson at 12.30, Dr. Minnitt in the afternoon and of course Mr. Watson-Jones at 5 p.m. I called to see Miss Taylor of <u>Philip, Son and Nephew</u>, 7 White-chapel. She gave me her awful experiences of the blitzes, and said she was very anxious to do all she can to push our publications.

After being driven to <u>Mr. Watson-Jones</u>' home to be there by 5 p.m prompt, I was shown into the waiting room, in which there were ten patients waiting to see Mr. Watson-Jones. He kept me waiting there until 20 minutes past 6. One of his assistants came in to settle up with one of his private patients who wanted to pay for her consultation and she blithely asked for three guineas [£3 3s/-]. Watson-Jones must be making a mint if he can make thirty guineas in a little over an hour.

Lord Reginald Watson-Jones[18] was full of vim and readily devoured all the suggestions I had to offer him for improvements on his new edition, and he has taken a note of these, which were a section on Physiotherapy, Possible Complications, Exercises after various Fractures and Rehabilitation. Regarding the new third edition of his book, there will be the following:-

(1)   A considerable amount of alteration and many new colour illustrations added.

(2)   I explained to him the difficulties with printing, binding, paper, and therefore there would likely be a lot of delays, and I encouraged him to make as much progress as is possible. I would like to start his new edition as soon as he can give me any material, but stressed that the latest date for making a start should be 1st January, 1942.

(3)   He wanted to know how long the present stock would last, and I retorted, "Could he tell me how long the war would last?" After explaining the difficul-

---

18 It seems Macmillan was dazzled by the great man. Watson-Jones was never a lord, though he was knighted in 1945.

ties in trying to give an accurate estimate, we decided that we should aim at getting the new edition out for June 1942.

Mr Watson-Jones was greatly interested in Brittain's book on arthrodesis. He thinks some of his illustrations are marvellous, and the operations ingenious. He says he must get a copy of this work as soon as ready.

Then like a bolt from the blue, he asked me what about this British Textbook of Orthopaedics!! I explained to him that since Nobby Clarke was in the R.A.F., Professor Platt had great difficulty in making progress.

He stated that one of the difficulties in having a book on fractures which was an outstanding success, was that he was becoming known as a Fracture Expert. He wants to contradict this statement and let everyone know that he is not a fracture expert but rather an orthopaedic surgeon, and fractures is only a small part of an orthopaedic surgeon's work.

He imagined that the best way to counteract this idea, was to do another companion book on Orthopaedic Surgery, but I reminded him that he was up to the neck in work, and although he had the printed sheets of the new edition in his possession for nearly six months, he had done no work on these at all. Therefore how could he possibly hope in such circumstances to write a new book on Orthopaedics and also keep it up to date? He agreed he could not do it meantime, but said that some day he was determined to do so.

I explained to him that what 1 really wanted was that he should do a section in this British Textbook on Orthopaedics. He maintains tha if he is to take part in this at all, then he must be one of the directors in the volume and not fourth from the bottom.

After Watson-Jones interview, I went along to Walton Hospital, and met most of the twenty-one doctors there in the Residency. This is the the place where you get all the secrets about your books, and these young doctors were very ready to talk about a variety of subjects which I have carefully made a note of for future reference...

I stayed the evening with my friend, Dr. Wyse, and about 9.30 I phoned <u>Professor Platt</u> at his private address. He was exceptionally nice to me on the telephone and informed me that he had spent the previous weekend with Professor Seddon at Oxford. When I asked him about the progress he was making with the Textbook of Orthopaedics, he said that he had given it further thought, was making plans for its development and laying a sure and solid foundation, but as he had so much work for the Government, organising the Medical Services, etc., he had not the time to devote to this publication which he would like.

On Wednesday morning, I left with the express train from Manchester to London. I arrived in at Euston at 2.20 and got in touch with Mr. Handfield-Jones' secretary who had arranged an appointment for me at 3.30 that afternoon. As I was entering 149 Harley Street, I ran right into Mr. Hamilton Bailey. He did not recognise me at first, said it was my bowler hat that was responsible for my changed appearance and said he had left full instructions with his secretary and was looking forward to my visit with great delight...

After my interview with Mr. Handfield-Jones, I found <u>Mr. Hamilton Bailey's</u> secretary. She gave me instructions how to get to his home and advised me to have tea, in town. I was instructed to take the tube to Totteridge, which is a three quarters of an hour journey from Tottenham Court Road. This will give you an idea how far out Mr. Hamilton Bailey stays from the centre of London.

Totteridge is one of the select suburbs in London; a few influential people have bought up all the ground, and according to Mrs. Hamilton Bailey the cheapest acre of ground costs £1,750. This ensures that no jerry built or small houses will be built in this suburb and Mr.

Hamilton Bailey's own home is an extremely beautiful one. His grounds occupy 6 acres and they have everything there – fruit trees, rose gardens, private swimming pool, vineries, etc. Mr. Hamilton Bailey lives out of doors all the year round. He has a hut designed for patients suffering from tuberculosis. This type of hut can be turned about to shelter from winds and rain and storm, and at the same time gives you the benefit of basking in the sunshine. I do not think however that he is long enough in the hut to take advantage of its comforts, as he retires to bed at 11 p.m. and is up every morning at 5.30 at the latest. Summer or winter, he has a dip in his private swimming pool, does his physical jerks in the open air, has a large medicine ball which he throws at anyone who will share in the fun with him, and keeps himself mentally and physically fit.

His home is luxuriously furnished. I do not think I have ever been in a bedroom with such lavish furniture. A small midget wireless set is at your bedside and every comfort conceivable. In his library he has a tremendous number of volumes, and I noticed he had all the up to date books, such as Nelson's Loose Leaf on Surgery and Medicine and all the other books which mean so much and indicate that he spares no expense in keeping himself up to date. He works continually by means of the dictaphone and I observed that he is always about a dozen or so records in advance, so that his secretaries are kept fully occupied.

I do not know if his chair is specially built for giving messages by dictaphone, but it is placed in the centre of the room, surrounded by tables, desks and chairs, etc., and when he mounts this large chair which is raised from the ground by about 18 inches, it is just like a king ascending the throne. Mr. Hamilton Bailey is over 6 ft. tall and his bulky dimensions fill this huge throne admirably.

Macmillan made a list of the subjects they discussed; of interest here, among the chapters proposed for revision, were Shock;

Anaesthetising the Wounded; Plasma Transfusion; and Injuries to Peripheral Nerves. He suggested that Hamilton Bailey might invite Seddon to contribute to the new edition.

> We talked on till 11.15. At the dinner time, a rather amusing incident occurred. He was explaining to me his difficulties with John Wright & Son, Publishers of Bristol. He maintains that if they had gone to their building after the blitz and had given those in charge of the building a £5 note, they would have brought out of the strong room any important documents they wanted. This means that they would have got over 2,000 of Mr. Hamilton Bailey's originals, but he had no doubt at all that Mr. John S. Wright would consider this most dishonest, and therefore they were left under water for six weeks, with the result that most of his originals were all spoilt. This trouble is aggravated because they advised him to prepare new drawings for all his illustrations, and sometimes he works a whole week on one particular drawing, then back comes word from Wright that they have found the original block and that it is in quite good condition.
> Mr. Hamilton Bailey warmed up as he explained, "You see, the annoying feature is this, that he belongs to that terrible sect the Plymouth Brethren," and the poor old P.B.s had a rough passage. Mrs. Hamilton Bailey retorted, "Hamilton, don't be so rash; what would you say if Mr. Macmillan was identified with this particular set of people?" I can still hear him chuckle "Not at all; he is far too level headed and sensible for such a thing; I know that by his letters." There and then I had humbly to confess that I had taken my place with these despised people. Mrs. Hamilton Bailey enjoyed the joke, and I think she giggled for nearly five minutes afterwards while Mr. Hamilton Bailey looked rather discomfited.

Macmillan visited more authors before continuing to Oxford.

Friday morning, I got the train leaving Paddington shortly after 9 a.m., came off at Reading and tried to make contact with the <u>Paper Control</u>. There were three persons in front of me to see Mr. Spring who looks after the boards, and there were many more waiting after I came out. He therefore only gave me 10 minutes for my interview.

I made the most of my time and rather impressed him with the importance of our publications. I explained to him that I had received word from Professor Seddon to come and see him about publishing a new book. What was the use of entertaining such an idea if, after we had the book all printed, we could not get boards for binding? Knowing the activities of Wingfield Morris Hospital and the good work that Professor Seddon and his team of experts are doing, he listened sympathetically to all I had to say. He would do his utmost to help us in our determined effort to obtain boards. The present position was extremely difficult but he had hopes that the position would not be so acute in the near future.

Later I travelled on to Oxford, called in to see Blackwells. Grant is away, and therefore I asked to see the man in charge of the Medical Section. He was out for lunch and would not be back till after 2 p.m. Wingfield Morris is about four miles out in the country and therefore it took me a good half hour to get there.

<u>Professor Seddon</u> is extremely nice. A young man, he cannot be any more than 36 to 40 years of age. His father knows some of my friends who are in Edinburgh, and as I mentioned that I was intimate with some of his relations, this helped to form a personal link.

Seddon also came from a family of Plymouth Brethren and this may explain the link with Macmillan and his family. Seddon rebelled from the rather strict way of life, but remained a committed Christian. Both he and Macmillan enjoyed finding apt biblical verses that, with a bit of editing, could be dropped into the conversation.

One of Macmillan's favourites was "Put not your trust in prin*ters*".

> The work he intends to publish is a special monograph
> about half the size of Watson-Jones' book on Fractures.
> It is dealing with Peripheral Nerve Injuries. They have
> a most ingenious method of dealing with these. Just
> now the hospital is full of wounded soldiers and airmen.
> If any part of the body shows loss of sensation due to
> injured nerves, that part of the body is clearly marked
> and a photograph taken. At operation, the actual nerve
> is exposed and again an accurate photograph is taken.
> There is a careful follow up of each individual case, and
> sometimes they have as many as 40 or 50 photographs
> taken before the case is actually finished with, and
> sometimes it takes a year or two before they are dis-
> charged.

Attempts had been made to suture nerves from the time of
the American Civil War onwards. In Europe the pioneer was
Theodor Kocher in Berne, Switzerland,[19] who was described by the
visiting Scottish surgeon Harold Stiles as "the most progressive surgeon of his generation". His methods were described in a *Textbook of
Operative Surgery*,[20] which would have been known to surgeons working at the wartime hospital at Bangour outside Edinburgh in the First
World War. Stiles also visited Harvey Cushing in America and so had
an international knowledge of surgical progress. Seddon would have
known of Stiles' work and probably owned a copy of his textbook.[21]
Macmillan spent some time with Seddon.

> An accurate filing system is kept of every case treated
> in the hospital, and he let me look over all his files. It is
> marvellous how accurately everything is detailed. He
> showed me one or two continental works on this and
> said that there is a great lack of such knowledge in the
> surgical profession at the present time.
>   He was extremely modest and wanted to know if
> Messrs. E. & S. Livingstone would publish the book for
> him. He would be responsible for the frame work, and I

---

19 Jellinek 1998.
20 Kocher 1911.
21 Stiles and Forrester Brown 1922.

think five or six other contributors will take part in the compilation of the book. When I said we would gladly undertake the publication of such a work, he said, "This is most kind of you to say so."

I felt it was too premature to go into details about finance, as Professor Seddon said it would take them about two years to complete the work. I did however roughly go over the usual financial details about royalty, 50/50 basis or publishing the work on commission basis. He said that all who were taking part did not want much out of the book and they were also prepared to spend some money on its production. What they wanted was a first class job made of it.

He was so pointed about the literature of the present day that I asked him what he thought of Mr. Souttar's article in "War Surgery". Quite frankly, he said that it was frightfully done – appallingly bad. I asked him whether or not he would write a section, if Mr. Hamilton Bailey approached him. He replied that as this was most important work at the present time he felt it was his duty to do so and would therefore gladly undertake the task. I think however he was under the impression that Mr. Souttar's article would be scrapped altogether and that he would do a new section to take its place. I have therefore reported this matter to Mr. Hamilton Bailey and am leaving it with him to put things right.

He was tremendously impressed with the production of "War Surgery". He said that he had never seen a more beautiful book in his life and assured me that as long as I was with E. & S. Livingstone everything he published would be done by them.

According to Professor Platt of Manchester, Seddon has the best orthopaedic brains in the country and will most certainly do some valuable work, and therefore I tried to press home the claims of the British Textbook of Orthopaedics.

I explained to him about Mr. Watson-Jones, how he was determined to do another companion book on

Orthopaedic Surgery, which Seddon believes he could easily do and make a splendid job of too. He therefore listened intently to all I had to say to him. I suggested that I should send him the preliminary arrangement that Professor Illingworth made for his "Textbook of Surgical Treatment" and promised to send him these two documents, one giving particulars about the editorial work and the second giving a detailed contents of the entire work. He said that he would endeavour to draw up similar documents for the proposed Textbook of Orthopaedics and write forcibly to Professor Platt. I asked him if Professor Platt had mentioned the book when he was staying with him during the previous weekend, but evidently it was never mentioned. Professor Seddon is extremely friendly, and I am sure he will be a good friend to our firm.

I left Wingfield Morris Hospital at 5 minutes past 4, and by a stroke of good luck managed to get into Oxford Station just as the train for Paddington was leaving. I had to stand for two hours journey from Oxford to Paddington and did not get in there until 6.30 p.m. After collecting my cases, I travelled home over-night with train from Kings Cross. The travelling on the train during this journey was not too bad, and only on one occasion, from Oxford to Paddington, was the train unduly crowded.

After arriving home, there are one or two things which seem to impress me most forcibly.

(1) The great damage that has been done to our cities, such as Manchester, Liverpool and London, and yet the determination of the people to carry on in spite of their heavy losses, is unforgettable. Let me illustrate this point; while in Liverpool I visited the old couple with whom I used to stay. Pop is aged 84 and Mop is about 75. The houses on each side of them were completely wrecked; they have a ten apartment home, and yet they can only use four rooms. Their front windows are blown in and they have that white gauze on the remaining windows, but there was Pop busily engaged in making

"Victory Vs." He tells me that he has already made about two gross.

(2) The second impression is this, that I cannot understand why Edinburgh has so far escaped, because we seem to be the only large city in Britain that has not suffered serious damage.

(3) The Medical Profession everywhere is most favourably impressed with the work we are doing at the present time, and therefore we should with gratitude do all we can to push forward the production of beautiful medical books which will help in the national effort at the present time.

Chapter 3

A professor in wartime: the Peripheral Nerve Injury Unit

Now it may not be immediately apparent why in those days orthopaedic surgeons – originally specialists in childhood injuries and diseases – should have the responsibility for making repairs to the nervous system, or indeed the expertise to do so. This is how Seddon explained it:

> The wound that injures a nerve often damages neighbouring structures – bones, joints, blood vessels and tendons – and it is, therefore, desirable that the surgeon choosing (or in times of war ordered) to devote himself particularly to the surgery of the peripheral nerves should have a wide range of skills. Moreover, reconstructive operations are sometimes necessary if a nerve cannot be mended or fails to recover satisfactorily after repair.

In practice, surgeons specialising in orthopaedics took charge of many aspects of a patient's treatment and so developed a range of different skills. Seddon also held strong views on patient management:

> As in the case of traumatic paraplegia – in which diverse skills are also required – the organisation should be such that the patient is never in doubt about who is looking after him. And as in some other disorders of the locomotor system a precise programme of treatment is all-important: the man who draws it up is the one to whom the patient knows he belongs. Moreover the commitment has no time limit. Ideally, the arrangements should be immune from disruption by administrative machinery. In Britain, during the Second World War, great pains were taken to ensure that this

was so; and despite the hazards of war and the dictates of geography, continuity of treatment and supervision was very good.[22]

When Seddon arrived in Oxford, he set about filling gaps in his knowledge of the physiology of peripheral nerve injuries by discussing the subject with JZ Young (discoverer of the squid giant axon and giant synapse) in the Zoology Department of the university, who forthwith reviewed the literature and found it deficient in solutions to the problems.[23] Young set up a unit funded by the Rockefeller Foundation to study nerve regeneration in mammals. His work, and that of other brilliant members of the unit, was of great importance to the repair of peripheral nerves.[24] One of the young zoologists was Peter Medawar, who became a Nobel Laureate as a result of his work on tissue grafts. For Seddon, it was a contribution Medawar made on the use of fibrin as a glue to help join nerves that was important.[25]

The race was on to marry scientific data with surgery to bring back useful life to shattered limbs in the hundreds of cases of nerve injury that were seen by Seddon and his Oxford staff. New scientific terms were needed to describe the different types of injury. The first type was when the nerve was completely severed, the second when the outer part was damaged but not completely cut and the parts of the nerve called the axons that transmit the signal still had some supporting tissue. The third case occurred when the damage only caused temporary paralysis and recovery did not involve the slow regrowth of the nerve. This is better described in Seddon's own words:

---

22 Preface to Seddon 1972.
23 Young 1942.
24 Seddon, Medawar and Smith 1943; Seddon, Young and Holmes 1942.
25 Seddon and Medawar 1942.

At a meeting of the Association of Physicians held in April 1941, I propounded the following classification:

1. Complete anatomical division of a nerve.
2. A "lesion in continuity," in which more or less of the supporting structure of the nerve is preserved but there is nevertheless such disturbance of the nerve fibres that true Wallerian degeneration occurs peripherally.
3."Transient block." – A minimal lesion producing paralysis that is incomplete more often than not; it is unaccompanied by peripheral degeneration and recovers rapidly and completely.

These three syndromes are well known to neurologists, and discussion centred chiefly on terminology. It may be argued with justification that "lesion in continuity" is ambiguous and might well include "transient block"; for there is no doubt that in transient block the nerve is in continuity. It was therefore suggested by Prof. Henry Cohen that distinctive names should be given to these three types of nerve injury so that confusion might be avoided.

The three terms – neurotmesis, axontmesis and neurapraxia – are now standard definitions and part of the English language. Although Henry Cohen actually coined them, it was Seddon who first saw the need for them and insisted they should come from Greek. He now had three new words to use in the book he was to write for E & S Livingstone. Cohen had gained first-class honours in 1922 and MD with special merit in 1924. He wrote:

Etymologically these words indicate the ideas they are intended to convey, and they have not previously been used – so that the field for them is clear.
1. *Neurotmesis* (*tmesis*, a 'cutting', which implies a separation of related parts), which describes the state of a nerve that has been completely divided. The injury produces a lesion which is in every sense complete.

2. *Axonotmesis*: Here the essential lesion is damage to the nerve fibres of such severity that complete peripheral degeneration has followed; and yet the sheath and the more intimate supporting structures of the nerve have not been completely divided, which means that the nerve as a mass of tissue is still in continuity.
3. *Neurapraxia* (*apraxia*, 'non-action') is used to describe those cases in which there is a short-lived paralysis – so short that recovery could not possibly be explained in terms of regeneration.[26]

These classifications had been established by experiment. Seddon described the appearance of axontmesis in rabbits following firm squeezing of a nerve with fine, smooth-bladed forceps: "the immediate lesion is of striking appearance: the central and peripheral parts are united only by a fine ribbon of translucent connective tissue. The main substance of the nerve is broken and separated by an appreciable interval. Within a few minutes it flows together again, and the fine connecting ribbon is filled out so that the gap is no longer visible."[27]

Seddon described similar experiments that were performed with JZ Young on patients in whom part of a limb required amputation: "on several occasions patients have allowed us to crush or divide a nerve, in the part to be sacrificed, at an appropriate level before the final operation". The general pattern of the nerve was maintained: "the axons were completely interrupted and the conjugating tissue appeared to consist of collapsed endoneurial tubes. In all but one case the lesion had been allowed to proceed to some measure of regeneration; there was a noticeable absence of the axonal branching and criss crossing that are always found after suture".

Seddon and Young recognised that the integrity of the Schwann tubes provided important support for regeneration: "if, as we believe, the process of regeneration is a protoplasmic outflow from the central stump (Young JZ 1942), progress will be faster when the flow is confined to one main channel and not dissipated in many separate protoplasmic streams". It is the difference between

---

26 Seddon 1942a..
27 Seddon 1943a..

preservation and destruction of continuity that underlies the division of degenerative lesions between those with the potential for spontaneous recovery and those that will not recover unless action is taken.

Colonel Davis, Senior Consultant to the Chief Surgeon in the European Theatre of Operations of the US Army, remarked that "the records of the Wingfield Morris serve as models: not so elaborate that they would obstruct the care of the wounded but that they should be complete so that future military surgery would benefit from the study. This required unified direction which was never obtained". This is an interesting comment, bearing in mind that one of the aims of the Peripheral Nerve Injuries Committee of the Medical Research Council had been to address this problem. Even in war it had not, it seems, been possible to impose such regulation on the different centres. The excellence of Seddon's notes, which were never written retrospectively, made them the foundation for his book.

Surgeons from the United States used to visit and study the methods used in Seddon's unit when they were in Europe; after 1942, the American Hospital – The Churchill, just across the road from the Wingfield-Morris – was functioning, which made contact easy. Seddon's department was considered unique.[28] However, the Americans found the British set-up strange in that "the RAMC found it possible to make use of Professor Seddon without insisting that he be in uniform".[29] The situation was different in America, where there were military hospitals whose doctors and surgeons were all part of the armed services and not civilians. In Britain, cases could be seen by either military or civil doctors and nurses in either type of establishment.

Although many people from Oxford had left to join the forces, the gap was filled by people from other countries. Some were stationed there and some had arrived as refugees, swept ashore ahead of a bow wave of tyrannical persecution in Europe. One who became an important figure in Oxford, and in Seddon's working life, arrived in the wake of the Spanish Civil War. Dr Josep Trueta had become known as a Catalan supporter fighting against General Franco in the Spanish Civil War and as a surgeon whose methods had reduced the number of amputees.[30] His method was to immobilise

28 Spurling 1958.
29 Davis 1964.
30 Trueta 1939.

the bones of a compound fracture by putting the limb and adjacent joints in plaster after setting the bones and cleaning and dressing the wound. The plaster and dressings were left in place for 4–6 weeks. To the amazed disbelief of many, infection was controlled and so limbs were saved; any blood and pus drained away through the dressings and the plaster cast. (This was in the pre-antibiotic era, but the practice of immobilisation continued later; a window was cut in the plaster to allow dressings to be changed.)

In 1938, after Hitler's annexation of Austria (the *Anschluss*), the venue for the International Congress of Surgery was changed from Vienna to Brussels. At the conference, Trueta was warned that his life would be at risk if he returned to Spain. Aided by several English admirers, he and his wife fled to London. There he gave a lecture attended by Girdlestone, who was sufficiently impressed to find work for him in Oxford. In 1939 he persuaded Nuffield to provide funds, and the Oxford Regional Hospital Board invited Trueta to work at the Wingfield-Morris Hospital. He soon became an adviser to the Minister of Health, which allowed him to work without renewing his qualifications as other refugees had to do. He did have to learn English. He was registered as a foreigner allowed to practise in the UK in September 1942.

There was a small team in the Dunn Laboratory in Oxford exploring the possibilities of fighting infection with an antibacterial called penicillin. Ernest Chain was the biochemist responsible for its extraction and purification (after growing it on the largest dishes available: bedpans). Chain had come to England in 1933 as a refugee from Germany. Professor Howard Florey, the pathologist of the team, engaged Trueta to work on some of the animal studies of the compound. More help was urgently needed so, when a new Nuffield Research Fellow Charles Fletcher arrived in Professor Witts' department, Witts introduced him to Howard Florey who asked him to find a patient who could be given some of the tiny amount of precious penicillin.[31] They had so little of it that the urine of the trial patients had to be collected so the penicillin could be extracted and purified for reuse; Mrs Florey and her husband bicycled round the hospitals to do this. Because a smaller dose could be used on younger patients, some children were volunteered.

---

31 Fletcher 1984.

Some of the first patients anywhere to receive penicillin were treated at the Wingfield-Morris, where the staff saw with some excitement the results in critically ill patients. The effectiveness of the antibacterial was apparent, but there just was not enough of it. Florey and Norman Heatly were flown to America where the process of large-scale production of penicillin could be achieved and a commercial product created. Howard Florey and Ernest Chain were later awarded a Nobel Prize jointly with Alexander Fleming.

The small rumblings of research in Oxford became like an exploding volcano, so powerful was use of penicillin in curbing infection of wounds. The sooner a wound was healed, the sooner Seddon could operate on damaged nerves. Penicillin could be put in a wound or given by injection, but not taken orally at that time. The other antibacterial used during the war was a sulphonamide: sulphanilamide. It had first been used directly on wounds and later was available for oral administration. After D-day, casualties arrived at the Radcliffe with labels on their stretchers; red labels gave the time and dosage for sulphonamides, yellow for penicillin.

Returning to Trueta's method of treatment described above, and published in *The Principles and Practice of War Surgery*,[32] the plaster cast – which absorbed fluid from the wound and remained unchanged – would begin to smell foul. Seddon must have found this an affront to ward hygiene, so he and Florey devised smell-proof fabric bags that could be put over the plaster on an arm or leg. They were not very effective, and anyway could not be used on the trunk.[33] However, Trueta's methods were useful before antibiotics became available. Seddon recalled: "That Trueta arrived in this country in 1939 was a god-send; after a short-lived display of scepticism, we were converted to the 'closed-plaster' regimen".[34] In October 1940 the Orthopaedic Section of the RSM held a discussion on "closed plaster treatment of wounds in the light of recent experience". The bacteriologist Dr ETC Spooner was invited to follow the discussion with his investigations on this subject.[35]

---

32 Trueta 1943.
33 Seddon and Florey 1942.
34 James 1978.
35 ETC Spooner, not the originator of Spoonerisms, WA Spooner, but a relative.

Of course there were many refugees, but two more particularly should be mentioned. Ludwig Guttmann was a surgeon who obtained a visa for himself and his family to visit England from Germany and then contacted The Society for the Protection of Science and Learning. They arranged an invitation to Oxford, where he was helped by the Master of Balliol and worked with Cairns at the Radcliffe. His research on the neuroregulation of sweat glands was relevant to the assessment of nerve injury, so he and Seddon had frequent discussions.[36]

The work of another refugee with a similar name, Ernst Gutmann, was also important to Seddon. Ernst was a Czech doctor who had done some physiology in Prague. His wife had fled Czechoslovakia in 1939, but he had been conscripted by the Germans and ended up a prisoner-of-war camp on Boar's Hill. He came to JZ Young's department as a cleaner, but Young was able to make better use of him as a researcher. The subject of his PhD was "recovery of function after denervation in mammals". After the war he and his family returned home, where he helped survivors of Teresienstadt before continuing his career and becoming a professor.

Ludwig Guttmann had already had excellent training in Germany and gained considerable experience. This led to differences of opinion and Seddon was not alone in finding him unwilling to concede a point. Guttman's frustrations ended when he was registered to practise in November 1943 and was able to work independently. George Riddoch suggested he could start a centre for paraplegics in the hutted Emergency Medical Service hospital at Stoke Mandeville. They were a very neglected class of patient; it was thought that very little could be done to help them. Guttmann made an outstanding success there, giving the patients dignity. He organised sports activities for them at a time when it was very shocking to the public to see cripples doing normal sports, but it was tremendously satisfying for the disabled. Eventually he was able to found the Paraplegic Olympics, for which he received a knighthood.

Professor Girdlestone still visited the Wingfield-Morris Hospital daily. He also had patients at the Chipping Norton and District War Memorial Hospital. On the wards in Oxford, he played to the gallery and where there were children he was greeted with

---

36 Guttmann 1940.

whoops of delight. By contrast, Professor Seddon was greeted with silent respect as he coolly made his way round his patients. He treated each with kindness, and the penetrating gaze from his blue eyes missed nothing.

When Seddon arrived in Oxford, he and Trueta worked together to modernise the way things were done in the hospital. The ward round included the professor, junior surgeons and postgraduate students. All of them would gather at the foot of a patient's bed for a discussion about the patient; Girdlestone would give his opinion and perhaps snap a photo. Seddon realised how inappropriate some of the remarks were: they baffled the patients and made them anxious. Henceforth, he decided, the discussion would take place in a lecture theatre, where Girdlestone could and did still have his say. If a photograph was needed, it was taken by a professional medical photographer. Ruth Bowden described the conferences that were held three days a week at 8.30 a.m.

> These were a gruelling experience for the newly appointed housemen and assistants who were responsible for preparing and presenting the patients. As in a Court Martial, the most junior members gave their own diagnosis first. It brought home the truth of Johnson's quip that "when a man knows he is to be hanged in a fortnight, it concentrates his mind wonderfully". It always remained a challenge but the anguish soon drained away. It provided an excellent training, and 'Prof' wanted to know the opinions of all the members of his team, however junior. Once the preliminaries were over, the discussion between the giants began. [Trueta] had a genius for picking out a small discrepancy and like HJS he would discuss and argue from first principles. Neither of these men ever dissembled, they were never ashamed to confess to puzzlement or uncertainty. This revelation of the openness and genuine humility of good minds was one of the most formative elements in our postgraduate education. Treatment was always discussed and sometimes even planned in concert. Where divergence of opinion

remained, the surgeon in charge carried out his plan and reported back to some future meeting.

Seddon encouraged foreign surgeons to visit, but this could have its downside. On one occasion, an American visitor made the ward round extremely irksome for Seddon by dictating, at each bedside, the treatment he would give, quite oblivious of the irritation he was causing.

Soon after Seddon's arrival, Trueta moved to the new accident service at the Radcliffe Infirmary. He took charge when its chief, a Canadian, Jim Scott joined up. Friction between Seddon and Trueta perhaps started at this time, because although the Wingfield-Morris was short of staff the situation was even worse in the accident service. Trueta made unreasonable demands that Seddon send him surgeons. In the end the Canadians were able to send some young surgeons. Seddon also upset Trueta by complaining that his case notes were inadequate, echoes of First World War shortcomings already referred to in Chapter 1. In the foreword to his book on war surgery, dedicated to Girdlestone, Trueta thanked many colleagues and "HJ Seddon, to whom, as to the other friends I have named, I am glad to express my deep gratitude". However, there was to be more friction between the two men in later years.

In August 1942, hard lessons were learnt by the commanders of the Dieppe Raid; it was a disaster. Jagged, explosively destructive high-velocity projectiles killed and injured many of the mainly Canadian force. Colonel JA MacFarlane, consultant surgeon at the Canadian Military Headquarters, warned that "the medical services in any future amphibian operation could anticipate radial nerve paralysis in as many as 40 per cent of fractured humeri, and joint involvement in an almost equal percentage of compound fractures" unless tactics of greater surprise and dispersal were used.[37] Seddon would see many of these sort of casualties.

The Emergency Medical Service, foreseeing increased demand for beds for air-raid casualties and evacuees, had planned hutted extensions to the Wingfield-Morris Hospital. They also took land from the Warneford Hospital to extend the new Churchill Hospital. Two wards for 'crippled children' were sponsored by Young

---

37 Harrison 2004a.

America and the British War Relief Committee. There were also orthopaedic, general surgery and plastic surgery beds. Money for the Churchill came from the British War Relief Committee Incorporated of the United States of America, and in 1942 the American Hospital in Britain moved to the Churchill from Park Prewitt near Basingstoke in Hampshire. For the first six months of 1942 it was staffed half the time as 23rd General Hospital and then half the time as the 91st General Hospital. Elsewhere in Oxford, the Examination Schools became a military hospital and Oriel and Balliol colleges were occupied by the Intelligence Corps and Chatham House.

Chapter 4

A tragic event

Everywhere there were manpower shortages as able-bodied young men were called up to fight. This affected E & S Livingstone as much as the hospitals in Oxford, as staff joined the forces. While exemption from active war service was given to people in certain professions, when Charles Macmillan visited Oxford at the end of August 1942 he was unsure of his own position, as he explained:

> AM/NCM   27th August, 1942.
>
> Dear Professor Seddon,
>   I was sorry I missed you when I was visiting Oxford. I would like very much to have discussed with you your book on "Peripheral Nerve Injuries."
>   I met the Secretary of the Publishers' Association in London and he was informing me that he does not think I will have any difficulty in getting another six months' extension after January 1943 and if I am still doing important work perhaps a further extension after this. The only danger is that the Ministry of Labour might shift me to some industrial work where administrative abilities are necessary.
>   The point I wanted to raise with you was one which I am sure you are well familiar with, that is, Professor Learmonth at the University here is doing a lot of work in these Peripheral Nerve Injuries and I was wondering if it was possible to ask him to do some selected section of your book. You may consider that you want the work done entirely by your team in Oxford and that this suggestion is outwith the scope of your work altogether, but I merely make this for what it is worth and I would like to know your re-actions to it...
>   I trust you have had an enjoyable holiday as you have had your full share of war work and you richly deserve it.

With all Kind Regards,
Yours sincerely,
      pro E. & S. LIVINGSTONE,
         Charles Macmillan
          MANAGER.

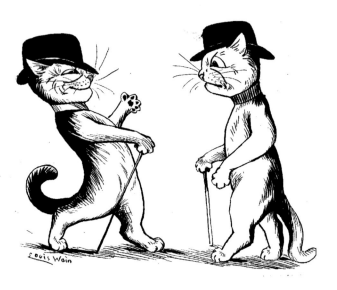

8. An unwelcome encounter; a cartoon by Louis Wain

Seddon was reluctant to work with this senior colleague and probably felt like the cat in the Louis Wain cartoon, so he replied diplomatically:

WINGFIELD-MORRIS ORTHOPAEDIC HOSPITAL
HEADINGTON
OXFORD
Telephone No .OXFORD 61151
31st August, 1942.

Dear Mr Macmillan,
I am relieved to hear that you have been given another six months' extension and seeing that you are always in

the habit of doing important work it looks as if there should be no difficulty about a further extension.

Professor Learmonth is a great friend of mine and I know what he is doing on peripheral nerve injuries. The idea of a combined effort is not unattractive but at the moment I do not see exactly how it would work out; I could explain this better if we could meet sometime for a talk. In case you do not happen to be in this part of the world in the near future it might help you to know that I expect to be in Glasgow on November 25th and 26th and, if it would not be troubling you too much, you might care to meet me at some convenient place there.

Although we are up to our necks in various investigations it might perhaps be well for us to put up a scaffolding for the book. Mr Highet is going into the Army and I suppose he will be comparatively unoccupied for a considerable part of his time, though ultimately he is expecting to do the nerve injury work for the M.E.F. However it ought to be possible for him to get on with certain sections of the book that would be peculiarly his own.

Yours sincerely,

H J Seddon

At the hospital William (Brem) Highet was assistant to 'Jim' Seddon, who had seen that he was a man "of some experience and enterprise" and found funds for his appointment a couple of years earlier to work at the Wingfield-Morris Hospital and to demonstrate anatomy in Professor Le Gros Clark's department. There were some exciting prospects of getting nerves in damaged limbs repaired more effectively than before, and there was so much work that Brem now worked full-time on this. All the data on the patients, the surgery and the results had to be carefully collected and analysed.

Sunday was a quieter day on the wards, and Brem would see his patients on this day accompanied by his three-year-old daughter Libby, who would chat to them and tidy their lockers, which they, of course, deliberately untidied in eager expectation of the visit. Calm reigned when the doctors did their rounds, but the nurses had to cope with all sorts of escapades from the high-spirited young men. Whether from the shortage of more usual materials or for other reasons, the patients made her a dolls' house of plaster of Paris, which she treasured. Perhaps it was not quite what the government had in mind when they said 'Make do and mend'.[38]

Certainly there were shortages, and the lack of raw materials to make paper resulted in a rise in price of such products. On 7 August 1942 the price of *The Times* was raised from 2d. to 3d. (three old pence), owing to the increased price of paper. Shortages of materials – such as the boards for bindings that Macmillan was concerned about when he went to see Paper Control in Reading, on his way to Oxford – affected E & S Livingstone and other medical publishers. They were trying to meet the demand of surgeons who needed to know the latest methods of treating war injuries.

After the Battle of Britain, one danger had passed, at least for the moment, and Oxford bells rang out to announce the victory. In Scotland, Macmillan was completing the production of Professor Illingworth's book and wrote to Seddon that:

> In going over the proofs of his new book, on coming to the chapters dealing with Peripheral Nerve Injuries, I mentioned that I hoped he had followed your system carefully. Professor Illingworth then told me that you were coming through as his guest on November 25th and 26th. The purpose of this letter therefore is to say that you might be as well to wait until you get to Glasgow before making arrangements for me to go through and see you ... With kind regards.

After meeting Seddon again, Macmillan wrote with optimism:

> I counted it as a great pleasure and privilege to meet you last Thursday the 26th ult. in Glasgow and I really think that we will be fortunate one day to have a really good monograph dealing with Peripheral Nerve Injuries. I will keep the information you have given me about the book in the meantime and I trust you will make all

---

38 Highet 2005.

arrangements possible so that we should attempt to publish the first edition towards the end of 1943.

I have also pleasure in sending you a draft of the formal agreement for your consideration. I can assure you that this agreement is drawn up on the usual lines and is recommended as the standard agreement by the Publishers' Association. As W. B. Hyatt, Esq., is now serving in Africa, I thought the best plan would be to leave him out of the agreement altogether. From your remarks I understand that you want his name to appear on the title page, but the names of the other three contributors will merely appear at the beginning of the chapters for which they are responsible. The fees we decide to pay them can easily be arranged at a later date.

I have prepared the agreement to cause you as little concern as possible and I therefore hope it will meet with your approval. If, however, you have you have any suggestions or additions to make, do not hesitate to let me know your wishes.

I also hope you had an opportunity of discussing the financial arrangements with Professor Illingworth before you left Glasgow.

If the draft agreement meets with your approval, then I will arrange to have this typed out in final form for signature and this will complete our preliminary arrangements.

I would like to have the opportunity of discussing further with you the proposed book on Orthopaedics as I have to meet Mr. Lambrinudi next Friday in London. If there are any things you would like to discuss with me when I am in London, which will be from the 8th to the 12th instant, I should be quite happy to come through to Oxford to see you, but as I explained to you in Glasgow I am frequently called down to London and if you have anything to discuss with me at any time I shall be pleased to come and see you in Oxford.

By "WB Hyatt" Macmillan meant Brem Highet. Constantine Lambrinudi had worked at a clinic in east London where he devised an ingenious operation for dropped foot.[39] Now 52 and a prominent orthopaedic surgeon, he was working at Guys Hospital. He had been considered a possible candidate for the chair at Oxford but was in poor health.[40] He died the next year of a coronary thrombosis.[41]

At the beginning of December Seddon was having doubts about being able to write a book so soon.

> Dear Mr. Macmillan,
> Since I returned from Glasgow I have been thinking about our proposed book and am now quite sure that it ought not to be completed before May or June 1944. This conclusion is reached after reviewing our material. Numerically, the number of cases is already adequate but when you consider that the full story of a case (leaving out of consideration the late end-result) is rarely completed in less than two-and-a-half years you will understand the need for delay. Two papers that were half prepared have had to be scrapped because of further information that compelled us to modify the conclusions reached in the early part of this work. Of course, there is no finality in anything scientific and a book can always appear in a Second Edition. But we must start with a pretty solid basis, and I think we shall have this by the end of 1943, and so be able to complete the book by the middle of 1944.
> I must warn you about one thing, As you know, I am responsible for a very busy Department. We have lost two of our most valuable men, one to the Air Force, the other to the Army, and there is an increasingly heavy burden of routine work. In this respect my position compares unfavourably with that of, say, Watson-Jones or Hamilton Bailey. If things get no worse than they are at present then this book can be done. But if they take away more people the position will be a desperate one so that even our war-time research may have to go. At

---

39 Fitzgerald and Seddon 1937.
40 Letter from D. Veale to Goodenough, University of Oxford Archives File UR6/MD/13/8.
41 Rocyn Jones 1956.

the present time I am working to the limits of what is physically possible. If I have to do more routine hospital work then something must go and the book, I am afraid, would have to wait. However, we must hope that this will not happen.

I am interested to hear that you will be seeing Mr. Lambrinudi next Friday; he is coming to stay with me on Tuesday, Wednesday and Thursday, and perhaps he will talk about the proposed book on Orthopaedics. There is, I am afraid, nothing we can do about the big book. I think Professor Platt has got his hands full with other things and his would-be collaborators are equally heavily engaged.

So far as I can see this draft agreement is very satisfactory and I would suggest you go ahead with the preparation of the final document.

Seddon was also working hard on a lengthy review that would be published in 1943: 'Three types of nerve injury'.[42] In it he highlighted the new terms axonotmesis, neurotmesis and neurapraxia "that have proved useful in a number of works in both clinical and experimental investigations". Using this classification he described methods of investigation of injuries, and reviewed clinical cases and experimental work from the huge amount of data that was accumulating as a result of the war. He consulted JZ Young and George Riddoch on the draft and gratefully accepted their suggested revisions. He also wrote on 'Peripheral nerves' for the *British Medical Bulletin*.[43] This was all very well, but Charles Macmillan was getting impatient for some sign of the book to be written for E & S Livingstone.

CM/FH   7th. December, 1942

Dear Professor Seddon
    Thank you for your letter of 5th inst. and I note that you now consider that your book on Peripheral Nerve Injuries should be delayed until May or June, 1944.
    We are always willing to be guided by our Author in

---

42 Seddon 1943a.
43 Seddon 1943b.

this direction, and I should like you to feel there will always be friendly co-operation and that you will not find us hard task masters.

I can well imagine that ideas regarding certain aspects of Peripheral Nerve Injuries must necessitate change from time to time, and there is always a right time to publish a work. This does not necessarily mean that we have to wait until all the advances are established, otherwise we would never publish any books whatsoever. I will therefore be quite happy to be guided by you regarding the date of publication of your work.

I also see that you are, like the most of us, heavily involved, and I know that organising and leading your Department is no easy task, but again we must act as circumstances will permit.

After I have seen Mr. Lambrinudi I purpose going home via Manchester and will endeavour to see Professor Harry Platt. I want to have a talk with him about the position of our proposed Textbook on Orthopaedics, and I will let you know the result of my interview at a later date.

As you have agreed to accept the terms of our Agreement, I have pleasure in sending you copies made out in final form, for signature. Attached to these, there is the usual List of Instructions for completing the Agreement. Will you be good enough to return all these documents to me as soon as you have signed them and had them witnessed.

No-one could have foreseen the disaster that was about to happen:

12th January, 1943.
Dear Mr. Macmillan,
A most tragic thing has happened. A few days ago we received news that W.B. Highet had been missing at sea since December 7th; he was on his way to South Africa to start a military Peripheral Nerve Injuries Centre.

There is, perhaps, some chance of his survival but the thing that concerns you is that he had in his possession a great deal of the material for the book on Nerve Injuries.

The case records on which this work was based are, of course, still here and the analysis of these cases can be done over again. But it will mean weeks, perhaps several months, of extra work and it is utterly impossible for me to tackle it all myself; there are not enough hours in the day. The man who succeeded Mr. Highet here is very good but not yet sufficiently experienced to understand what is involved.

I am afraid therefore that delay in the completion of the book is quite inevitable, though until I have gone into all that Highet was doing I cannot give you an estimate of the extra time that will be needed.

Of course Macmillan could only sympathise:

CM/FH   15th January 1943

Dear Professor Seddon,
Your letter of the 12th. inst. stirred me strangely. It is, undoubtedly, a terrible tragedy, and I can only hope the worst has not happened. I quite sympathise with you in this severe loss which you have sustained, and it will make the writing of Peripheral Nerve Injuries very difficult for you.

As far as obligations to the firm are concerned, I would not wish you to be anxious about those in the slightest. our mission in life is merely to be of service to the Medical Profession, and although a contract is signed and a working understanding reached, you will always find us most sympathetic in such trying circumstances as you mention in your letter.

Only last week, Mr Watson-Jones was praising the abilities of Dr. W. B. Highet and he has helped him a lot in the Chapter dealing with Vascular Injuries in his New Third Edition of Fractures.

All I can say meantime is that I hope we shall hear better news in the future.

As far as your own book is concerned, I would not like you to feel anxious in the slightest degree, although I am still hopeful that one day we shall have the pleasure of putting this book through the Press for you.

Brem Highet had boarded the SS *Ceramic* at Liverpool along with 600 others, mainly medical and nursing staff. On 6 December, shortly before midnight, the ship was hit by a torpedo. Only one survivor was picked up (as a witness) and made a prisoner of war. In a summary tribute, Watson-Jones wrote of "a brilliant young surgeon of engaging personality whose clinical ability, operative skill and scientific achievement have been paid as one of the tragic costs of war. His full contribution had not been made".[44] Coates Milsom of Auckland, New Zealand, remembered the impact of his loss:

> The tragic death of W.B. Highet during the recent war cut short the promise of a New Zealander who in Oxford had already contributed valuable studies; in 1941 he won the Jacksonian prize for his essay Injuries to the Peripheral Nerves with Special Reference to the Late After-results, and his contributions to *The Lancet* (1942) and the *British Journal of Surgery* (1943) showed the quality of work that would have been maintained if he had lived.[45]

As well as the personal loss, Brem's widow had to survive without a pension and this she did by continuing to work as a nurse. Life for herself and for little Libby was hard. Brem Highet's abilities had ranged from the practical – for example, he invented a small but very useful electrical device coupled with a hypodermic syringe for identifying and injecting a nerve (Fig 10) – to the intellectual, as shown by further publications.[46]

Among the latter was a paper titled 'Effect of stretching

44 Watson-Jones 1943.
45 C Milsom 'The first half-century of orthopaedic surgery in New Zealand', *JBJS*, **32B** (1950) 4, pp. 611–614 at 612.
46 Highet and Holmes 1943, Highet and Sanders 1943.

nerves after suture'. If end-to-end suture of nerves was carried out when there was a large gap, the extreme position in which the joint had to be held immobile by traction damaged the nerve, however carefully the operation had been done. So other means were tried which did not put the joint in absurd positions. These were "wide exposure and mobilisation of the nerve, transposition of the nerve and bone shortening." but resulting function was still poor.[47] More success could be had in hand injuries, and Bunnell and Seddon showed that, in the case of digital nerves, where the gap was smaller than in the cases looked at by Highet, a method of autogenous nerve grafts could work. These were small nerves and there were other nerves that could be used for the graft, which was not so with the major nerves.[48] Over the years several more papers were published on the subject in Britain and the USA.[49] These examples show the complexity and diverse methods of nerve repair that Seddon would have to describe in his textbook.

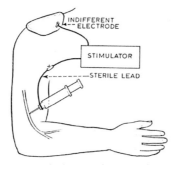

9. Fig 3.25 in *Surgery of Disorders of the Peripheral Nerves*. Highet's apparatus for nerve blocking. The needle is a stimulating electrode and is coated, except at its tip, with insulating resin.

In a letter of 19 May 1943, Macmillan urged Seddon:

> I am particularly anxious to know what progress you are making with your textbook on Peripheral Nerve Injuries, and being in the vicinity, I hope that it will be convenient for you to see me.
> I am just at the last stages now of the Third Edition of Mr Watson-Jones' Fractures and Joint Injuries, and I

---

47 Seddon and Riddoch 1953.
48 Seddon 1943b.
49 Seddon and Holmes 1944; Seddon 1954 (the Medical Research Council's Special Report); Seddon 1947c; see also Office of the Surgeon General, *Surgery in World War II*, 2 vols, Washington, DC, 1958–9.

WATSON-JONES. Fractures and Other Bone and Joint Injuries.

In the Press. By R. Watson-Jones, B.Sc., M.Ch.Orth., F.R.C.S.,
To be Hon. Orthopædic Surgeon, Liverpool Royal In-
Published firmary, and Robert Jones and Agnes Hunt Orthopædic
Shortly. Hospital ; Consulting Orthopædic Surgeon, Royal
Lancaster Infirmary, North Wales Sanatorium,
Birkenhead, Hoylake and
West Kirby, Wrexham
and East Denbighshire,
and Garston Hospitals ;
Clinical Lecturer in
Orthopædic Surgery and
Lecturer in the Pathology
of Orthopædic Conditions,
Liverpool University. A
Royal medium 8vo volume
of approximately 600 pp.,
containing about 1,000
illustrations, many of
which will be in colour.
(1939.)

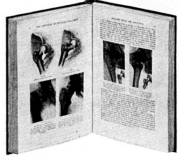

" This book is intended for
the practising surgeon and   (Size of Open Page, 9¾ × 6¾ inches.)
the senior or post-graduate
student. The general principles of fracture treatment are emphasised,
and details of technique profusely illustrated by photographs. Many
illustrations are in colour. Nerve injuries, vascular complications and
recent work on Volkmann's contracture are discussed. The section on
pathological fractures is illustrated by a complete series of radiographs
of bone tumours, infections and general skeletal diseases. The author's
work on fractures of the spine, dislocations of the pelvis and fracture
of the neck of the femur is included, together with new work on
avascular necrosis in bone and joint injuries, Perthe's coxa plana,
traumatic herniation of the intervertebral disc, and the treatment of
spondylolisthesis."—*Publisher's Note.*

10. Entry in the E & S Livingstone catalogue advertising
Watson-Jones book

observe that he pays your team at Oxford very high
praise in his Preface. He also makes reference to the
tragic loss of Mr. Bremner Highet, and I suppose this
grave loss will have hampered you in your progress.

I can assure you I am not trying to harass you in any
way, but being in the vicinity, I thought that at an interview, we could discuss quite freely, your new textbook.

Great care had been taken in the production of Watson-Jones' book, the third edition of *Fractures and Joint Injuries*. Macmillan ensured that the fibre of the pages would run in such a way that each page fell flat when the book was opened. In the preface to this edition, Watson-Jones remarked that copy had been "destroyed by the effects of fire and explosion; proofs have been delayed by the emergencies of casualty surgery" and he apologised that the book had been out of print for many months. He thanked E & S Livingstone and Charles Macmillan "for skill in surmounting obstacles, to the engravers, printers and binders for care and attention to detail". He also thanked "Professor Seddon and his team at Oxford for material on ischaemic contracture".

Seddon replied to Macmillan:

> I have an interesting suggestion to make to you about the book on Peripheral Nerve Injuries, but you will understand that progress has been hindered still further by my absence from the country since late February. I have only just returned from a Government mission that I had to undertake in Malta.

Seddon prepared his annual report for the academic year.[50] The "well equipped and, as we thought, commodious block provided by the generosity of Lord Nuffield" had become too small. They needed to update the X-ray and photographic departments; they needed more laboratories and a lecture theatre. Dr Branscombe Zachary replaced Brem Highet; Margaret Myers joined the nerve injuries team. Dr Ernst Gutmann continued his experimental work with a grant from the Fluid Research Fund and was also doing some clinical work and research with Ludwig Guttmann. Research work begun by Miss Smith was continued by Shirley Williams, and Mr FK Sanders was doing work in the Zoology Department on the traction of nerves. An electromyograph was being made for Ruth Bowden to use.

In the next year Seddon got a prefab to house the X-ray department, and the old X-ray space was converted for photography. However, Dr Fred Kemp (the radiologist) found the equipment,

---

50 Wingfield-Morris Hospital Annual Report 1943/4.

while adequate for clinical use, was not good enough for research. The Wingfield-Morris Hospital Committee opposed the building on their land of the laboratory and animal house that Seddon very much wanted. As for developing his teaching, the students had too much else in their course to fit in lectures about orthopaedic surgery. Seddon had set his sights on a creating a first-class university department and these frustrations were rumblings and grumblings of worse to come.

Chapter 5

Poliomyelitis in the colonies

From his pre-war work at the Royal National Orthopaedic Hospital in London and from patients in the Wingfield-Morris Hospital, where he was Clinical Director, Seddon had accumulated considerable knowledge of poliomyelitis and practical experience of treating patients.[51]

Poliomyelitis appears first as a fever and malaise with aches, particularly in the neck and back. The initial flu-like symptoms may be quickly followed by paralysis of arms or legs, or even of the muscles used to breathe. This is because the virus affects the nerve cells in the cervical spine, and occasionally the brain, that control movement. To be able to breathe, the patient sometimes had to be encased in a respirator – an 'iron lung' that enclosed most of the body. Eventually some recovery to muscle control could be expected, but often the muscles became wasted.[52]

In 1940–41 there was an epidemic of polio among British military personnel in Egypt, which came as a shock to all concerned, because this viral disease had not been recognised as common there; moreover, it was a disease that usually affected small children, not adults. Had it been brought in with the forces? News of the outbreak was suppressed at the time, but an account was published after the war by two of those who worked at the 15th Scottish Hospital in Cairo.[53] In the second year of the epidemic, 106 cases were diagnosed and 33 patients died. Six different strains of the virus were isolated at the 15th Scottish Hospital in Cairo.[54]

At the time of this unexpected outbreak in Egypt, the allies' success in the war in North Africa depended on their being able to use Malta as a base for attacks on shipping carrying supplies to the German and Italian troops. Years later, Joseph Galea recalled this stressful period:[55] "For two anxious years in 1941 and 1942 the fate

---

51 Seddon 1940.
52 Paul 1971.
53 Caughey and Porteous 1946.
54 Van Rooyen and Morgan 1943.
55 Galea 1952.

of the Second World War hinged on the defence of Malta. This little island situated in the centre of the Middle Sea possesses strategic value of the highest importance, and the Power that controls it dominates the flow of men and materials between three continents."

Ships bringing food were bombed or torpedoed, and serious food shortages resulted. The Maltese and the service personnel based there suffered daily bombing raids. Their air-raid shelters were caves under the island, where they had to endure most insanitary conditions. The polio outbreak in Egypt was matched by a similarly sized epidemic of typhoid fever on Malta, followed in 1942–3 by an epidemic of polio. Three of the 'four horses of the apocalypse' – war, pestilence and famine – had visited the island. Some supply ships of one convoy managed to reach the island in November 1942 and conditions began to improve. The health of the Maltese people and of the allied servicemen stationed there was crucial in defying the enemy forces in the Mediterranean.

Oliver Stanley was Colonial Secretary in the Churchill government, with a place in the Cabinet. He wrote for help to the Vice Chancellor of the University of Oxford, Sir David Ross.

Colonial Office
Downing Street
S.W.1.
12th February 1943

Dear Sir David

I am writing to you in connexion with a sharp outbreak of infantile paralysis which occurred recently in Malta. Starting at the end of November, the outbreak reached its peak in the middle of December and is now declining. There have been some 400 cases, of which about 10 per cent have been affected by severe paralysis.

During the epidemic Brigadier McAlpine, a consulting neurologist, serving in the Middle East, visited Malta and we have now received by telegraph his summary of the situation. He is satisfied with the measures that have been taken by the local civil medical authorities to prevent the spread of the disease and also with the treatment given to cases in the acute stage.

He considers that the treatment of the resulting paralysis is satisfactory in most cases but he indicates that the treatment is carried on in the face of certain difficulties. Brigadier McAlpine advises that a visit to Malta should be made by an orthopaedic surgeon.

Field Marshal Lord Gort, the Governor of Malta, who is at present in this country, had already suggested that a surgeon should be sent to deal with the rehabilitation of cases disabled by the disease.

After consultation with my Medical Adviser, who has discussed the matter with the Ministry of Health and with the War Office, I have decided that an Orthopaedic Surgeon should be sent to Malta by air at the earliest possible moment.

The Ministry of Health have suggested Mr. H. J. Seddon, F.R.C.S., Nuffield Professor of Orthopaedic Surgery. I am, accordingly,writing to you to ask whether it would be possible, if Mr. Seddon is willing, for his services to be lent to the Government of Malta for this mission. I am most fully aware that it will be difficult to release Mr. Seddon, even for a short period. I can only urge that the people of Malta, who after a weight of attack unprecedented in history, which they have endured with fortitude and loyalty, have claims which seem to me to be difficult to resist. This outbreak, which has attacked mainly children under five, has been a bitter blow to the Maltese at a time when they were beginning to emerge from a period of acute food shortage.

A period of one month has been mentioned as roughly the time to be spent in Malta but this and other details would be matters for discussion with the individual surgeon who is to go. If you see your way to release Mr. Seddon for this mission, it is proposed that he should continue to draw his normal emoluments which could, if desired, be paid during the mission by the Government of Malta. In addition, it is usual to pay a subsistence allowance to cover any additional expenditure that might be occasioned.

In view of the great urgency of the matter Mr Seddon has been informed informally that the request is being made. I should be much obliged if you would be so good as to let me have an immediate reply, by telegram if convenient. Arrangements could then be made to discuss with Mr. Seddon at once the details of the mission and to arrange an air passage for him at the earliest possible moment.

Yours sincerely

Oliver Stanley[56]

Seddon and Stanley both thought the request was one which they "could not possibly refuse, more particularly in view of the heroic part played in the war by the inhabitants of Malta". Seddon went to see Mr Miles at the Colonial Office. The university agreed to the financial arrangements, by which the Government of Malta would pay part of his salary while he was there. Rapid discussions took place between Seddon and the Governor, Field Marshall Viscount Gort, Lieutenant Governor Mr DC Campbell and those more directly involved: Major General LT Poole, Director of Pathology, Army Medical Service, Brigadier WK Morris DDMS, Malta, the government's Chief Medical Officer Professor AE Bernard, Professor TE Debono and the staff at St Luke's Hospital. Stanley wrote again to Sir David Ross on 19 February:

I understand he will have to take a Nursing Sister with him and a quantity of materials necessary for the treatment of his patients as well. The only way of reaching Malta at present is by air, and you can well imagine how heavy is the pressure on the available air space to the Western Mediterranean both for passengers and for freight at this time. I have, however, written to the Secretary of State for Air asking for his personal help in securing the facilities necessary for Professor Seddon's visit and I have every hope it will be possible to arrange for him to leave England next week.

56 Oxford University Archives FA6/13/1 annual report for Nuffield and CQ/11/8A/2.

I know well how important is the work in which Professor Seddon is engaged at Oxford. I am the more grateful to you for releasing him and to him for so readily undertaking what will, I fear, be a somewhat arduous mission. The people of Malta deserve the best that we can give them, and it is for that reason that I asked for his services.

Seddon arranged cover for himself during this mission through his contacts in the USA, and Major Kahn from the 298th General Hospital, University of Michigan, was assigned for temporary duty at the Wingfield-Morris. There was an ulterior motive in this because the US Army hoped to set up the 298th General Hospital in the UK as a peripheral nerve injury centre. In the end, this did not happen "because of the rule to hold injured in general hospitals not longer than than 180 days after admission: they were then to be returned to the United States".[57] The essential continuity of treatment was not possible in the UK.

Seddon left on 24 February 1943, only twelve days after the Colonial Secretary's letter, and was back in Oxford on 1 May. An aftercare nurse went out with him and stayed until August. By the time Seddon arrived, the epidemic of polio was waning and he could not find conclusive causes of the outbreak. In consultation with the Colonial Office and the Government of Malta, he made plans to establish a permanent physiotherapy department, an orthopaedic department and a system of clinics like those in England. In late May the vice chancellor of the university received a letter of appreciation of Professor Seddon's services from Oliver Stanley.

In 1944 the Vice Chancellor, who was also chairman of the Nuffield Committee, granted Seddon leave to make another visit to Malta. "If the RAF can take him he will go from 30th Dec to 18th January." Air transport had improved to such an extent that the journey there now took only about nine hours. Seddon was the first author of the report published in 1944 about the circumstances of the outbreak.[58] The first three points in his summary were these:

---

57 Davis L 1964.
58 Seddon, Agius, Bernstein and Tunbridge 1945.

1. During the period Nov 1942 to Feb 1943 there was an epidemic of anterior poliomyelitis in the islands of Malta and Gozo. There were 483 cases in all, 426 civilians and 57 men in the services.

2. The incidence fell most heavily on Maltese children under five years of age (82 per cent), 61 persons over the age of 20 years were affected, and of these only four were Maltese, the remainder, the service cases, being from the United Kingdom.

3. The mortality rate was high in the services (19.3 per cent) and low among the civilians (3.5 per cent +), the chief cause of death being respiratory paralysis.

In 1943 the US Army Epidemiological Board on Neurogenic Virus Diseases investigated the causes of unexpected poliomyelitis. Finally it discovered that the virus already existed in the area, but the local population obtained immunity when very young and there were rarely noticeable symptoms.[59]

January 1945 saw Seddon pay a return visit to Malta, coinciding with the publication in the *Quarterly Journal of Medicine* of his report on the polio epidemic. By this time a Maltese orthopaedic surgeon who had gained experience at the Wingfield-Morris was running an orthopaedic service in Malta. Seddon also read a paper at the Royal University of Malta on 'A short history of scrofula'. Scrofula is the old name for a presentation of tuberculosis as swellings on the neck. There was a superstitious belief that it could be cured by the touch of a king or queen.[60]

The management of poliomyelitis once again demanded Seddon's attention when in March 1945 there was an outbreak in another British colony, this time on Mauritius, off the coast of Africa. Oliver Stanley, still at the Colonial Office, sent a letter to the university, where Sir Richard Livingstone had replaced Sir David Ross as vice chancellor.

---

59 Paul 1971.
60 Seddon 1945a.

Your predecessor very generously came to our assistance in 1943. We are now faced with a serious outbreak in Mauritius, where the material damage done by hurricanes makes the danger of it assuming even more serious proportions a very real one.

After consultation with both the Ministry of Health and my Medical Advisers here, I feel that it is essential that we should get the best possible expert Adviser out to Mauritius at the earliest moment. The Ministry of Health have suggested that if it were possible for Professor Seddon again to be spared, the help he would give would be quite invaluable, and Sir Francis Fraser, the Director General of the Emergency Medical Service, has, I understand been in informal touch with Professor Seddon about this.

The Governor of Mauritius also welcomed expert advice and agreed to pay Seddon, who would also receive a pound a day subsistence. Seddon gave some advice on immediate measures to be taken and arranged to travel out to Mauritius.

Dr Alan M Macfarlan, an epidemiologist, was sent from the Emergency Public Health Laboratory, which was directed by the Medical Research Council. He and Seddon set out by air on 6 April with Constance Crossley from the massage department of the Wingfield-Morris Hospital. On the way, Seddon reported that "In Nairobi we recruited an Army pathologist and a medical officer in the Air Force, an old house officer of mine". All arrived on 15 April in Mauritius.

Patients were sought out and examined in every part of the island; we organised a hospital in some army huts erected on a race-course, and established a splint workshop at H.M. Prisons in Port Louis. Although the work was most strenuous we were greatly encouraged by the enthusiasm of many of the people in Mauritius. The nursing staff was almost wholly drawn from French Mauritius V.A.D.s who, after a short period of instruction, became most competent. The Chief Prisons

Officer, a jovial Irishman, was so successful in arousing the interest of his charges, some of them desperate criminals, that they not only made splints of the first quality, but spent such little spare time as they had making toys for the children in hospital.

Together with local experts they studied the epidemic, looking at the type of virus, how it could have been spread and so on. A report by McFarlan, Dick and Seddon was published in the *Quarterly Journal of Medicine*.[61] Donal Brooks commented:

> There his remarkable organising ability and enthusiasm enabled him to establish treatment centres with the help of the local doctors. Furthermore the physiotherapists, often working in difficult circumstances, were taught to record their observations on muscle charts, so that the information could be used later for clinical research. He also developed simple splints that could be made locally by ordinary craftsmen and which proved very valuable in the prevention of deformity.[62]

This type of splint was used elsewhere afterwards and referred to as 'the Mauritius splint'.

Seddon received generous hospitality in Mauritius among the French-speaking families with whom he was able to speak fluent French. He recommended that a young man that he met, Albert Menagé, should study medicine at Worcester College in Oxford. Mauritius was so refreshingly different and there were interesting scenes to photograph and later to paint (Fig 11). He found time to give a lecture on 'the private citizen and the public health'.[63]

The government and the Colonial Office agreed to establish an orthopaedic service and to send a British surgeon and two masseuses to the island in May. A Mauritian surgeon, Mr CA Bathurst, came over to train at the Wingfield-Morris and it was expected that he would be ready to return in two years. Initially he would work in Mauritius under Mr Fitton. Two technicians were trained at the Wingfield-Morris to supply appliances on the island.

---

61 McFarlan, Dick and Seddon 1946.
62 Brooks 1978.
63 Seddon 1945.

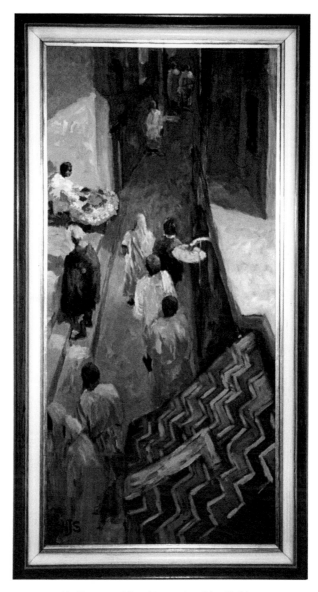

11. *Benares, Mauritius*, painted by Seddon

On 27 August the registrar of the university passed on a letter of appreciation from the Colonial Office:

> The work he has carried out in Mauritius on this occasion both for the immediate treatment of the victims, and in the advice he has given to the Government of Mauritius in regard to the aftercare of patients and the permanent organisation for the rehabilitation of cripples will be of the utmost benefit to that Colony. In addition, he is giving much valuable assistance since his return to this country in connection with a number of matters arising out of his visit to the island and to Kenya, particularly in regard to the establishment of orthopaedic institutions.
> Yours sincerely,
> G.H. Hall

Seddon replied to Douglas Veale, the registrar, who had started his career in the Civil Service, had risen quickly and then moved to become registrar at the University of Oxford. The various Nuffield benefactions were in part the result of his skill in steering vision into practicality. He could be found in the university offices in the Clarendon building, which became known as the 'hôtel de Veale'.[64]

> Dear Veale,
> I should become insufferably conceited had I not had some experience of the Colonial Office; they are so very polite and this is just their way of saying that I have not brought disgrace on the University. I shall never forget a conference at the Colonial Office when in the excitement of the moment I said that somebody "didn't care a damn" about something; they were horrified.
> Yours ever,
> H.J.S

---

64 *Oxford Dictionary of National Biography.*

Some of the surgical help that could be given to polio victims was remarkable. On one occasion Seddon brought back with him a boy whose legs and arms were so flexed that he could neither sit nor stand, but lay in a basket. After operations and physiotherapy, the boy was able to walk. Seeing so many patients with polio and treating them gave Seddon expertise and of course he published.[65]

In December there was an outbreak of polio in St Helena. This time, Seddon sent one of his former house officers from the Royal National Orthopaedic Hospital, now serving in the armed forces as Surgeon Lieutenant-Commander Karl Nissen. Early the next year, 1946, the problem was in Singapore and McFarlan went there.

Polio was not a disease confined to the colonies, because in 1947–8 an epidemic hit Britain. More research into prevention was needed. In 1949 the British Orthopaedic Association met in Bristol and Mr JM Fitton from the Floreal Hospital in Mauritius, after a brief reference to the geography, economy and races of Mauritius, described the orthopaedic service that had been developed since the time of their epidemic. In the discussion afterwards, Seddon referred to "the difficulty and magnitude of the task which Mr Fitton had so modestly described, and the fact that this individual's work often had to take second place to more pressing communal medical needs. Colonial orthopaedic centres had now been established in Malta, Nairobi and Lagos." He added that "it was imperative that the men who undertook this pioneer work should have the prospect of suitable places when they returned home".

On Seddon's death, the ambassador to Britain from Argentina remembered with admiration his high skill and devoted spiritual strength and modesty during a polio epidemic that occurred later in that country.

---

65 Seddon 1946b, 1947c, 1947d, 1948; Seddon, Hawes and Raffray 1946.

Chapter 6

Notable patients: the battle for life and recovery

Returning to the wartime challenges at home, Seddon wrote on 28 July 1943 to "J. McDonald Walker, Esq., D.F.C., Messrs. E & S Livingstone, 16-17 Teviot Place" as follows:

> Dear Mr. Walker,
>
> When I was away I prepared an outline for the book on Peripheral Nerve Injuries and as far as I can tell it will run to 35,000-40,000 words. If you could possibly allow it I would like to include about 150 illustrations (!), and two-thirds of them would be half-tones.
>
> I think you can count on the book having a good sale in America, but you would no doubt be taking this into consideration anyway.
>
> I happened to be spending my holiday with Liddell-Hart who is a writer of considerable distinction and abut twenty-five years' experience. I told him how much, or rather how little, spare time I have for writing and we reached the conclusion that, barring accidents, I ought to get the thing done by February. But it is just possible I may have to go to America, though I know nothing definite as yet. If I do so it would be to talk about Nerve Injuries – then there would be yet another delay. But I know what an understanding person you are; there is only one thing we can count on in wartime and that is the unexpected.
>
> Yours sincerely,
>
> H. J. Seddon.

His letter was acknowledged by the publishers. At a mere 40,000 words the book was considered quite short and Seddon could have as many illustrations as he wished. The publishers dangled another carrot to encourage him – good sales were expected in Australia, New Zealand and Canada as well – and they hinted "It would be excellent if we could have the whole manuscript complete by February and it is to be hoped that you will manage to do it in that time but of course we shall just have to leave it to you to do your best under circumstances."

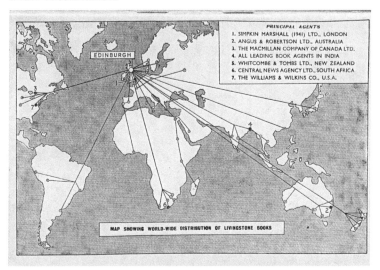

PRINCIPAL AGENTS
1. SIMPKIN MARSHALL (1941) LTD., LONDON
2. ANGUS & ROBERTSON LTD., AUSTRALIA
3. THE MACMILLAN COMPANY OF CANADA LTD.
4. ALL LEADING BOOK AGENTS IN INDIA
5. WHITCOMBE & TOMBS LTD., NEW ZEALAND
6. CENTRAL NEWS AGENCY LTD., SOUTH AFRICA
7. THE WILLIAMS & WILKINS CO., U.S.A.

MAP SHOWING WORLD-WIDE DISTRIBUTION OF LIVINGSTONE BOOKS

12. The geographical reach of E & S Livingstone as shown
on the back cover of their 1941 catalogue

Basil Liddell Hart was a military historian who had served in the First World War. He was a friend of TE Lawrence, Robert Graves and other writers. During the Second World War he moved to the peaceful landscape by the shores of Windermere. His second wife was the widow of a brilliant young chest surgeon, HP (Tim) Nelson, who had tragically died of infection following a diathermy needle injury. Nelson's career path had been similar to Seddon's in that he had worked at the RNOH in 1929 and 1930 as a registrar and gone to Ann Arbor on a scholarship the next year. When Nelson returned to England, a publisher from Churchills commissioned him to write a book for their Recent Advances series. It was unfinished when he died. One day in the future the names Churchill and Livingstone would be united, continuing the Recent Advances series.

The Nelsons and their two daughters were friends of the Seddons. There were other connections too, because Seddon had recently treated Basil Liddell Hart's son Adrian in Oxford, and Adrian was a patient at the same time as the commander of the 7th Armoured Division, John Harding, later Field Marshall Lord Harding of Petherton. The story of his injury and treatment illustrates a typical surgical case faced daily by Seddon.

John Harding had taken over command of the 7th Armoured Division on 14 September 1942 and during the battle of El Alamein in North Africa in October he was responsible for the division's break-out. Monty called him "that little tiger". He received a wound on 25 October, but continued to lead his division in the pursuit of Rommel and the German and Italian forces. In the engagement of 19 January, he was wounded severely.

According to his biographer Michael Carver, it was like this:[66] Harding was standing on top of a Grant tank looking through binoculars when a shell landed in front of the tank, killing one of the crew and hitting and wounding Harding, from his left arm across his body to his right leg. He sheltered under the tank until rescued. He probably was wearing neither tin hat nor battle dress, and his first conscious memory was of being angry at the doctor who cut off his new cavalry twill trousers. His life was in danger so he was transferred by air ambulance the next day to the casualty clearing station near Sirte, though the air ambulances were not usually allowed into forward positions.

John Harding spent three months in 63rd General Hospital in Cairo recovering from "a fractured right tibia, right radius and wrist, amputation of second third and fourth fingers, and penetrating wounds to the thigh, left chest wall and right arm" – those were the details he sent in a telegram to his wife. He was on the dangerously ill list until 17 February. In May he was fit enough to be sent home by flying-boat via Khartoum, Congo and West Africa. It was an arduous journey: three times a day he had to get in and out of the plane and he had to dress his wounds. He was graded D at a medical board near Bristol. His main problem was lack of movement in his lower left arm. He was sent to Jim Seddon, "who operated on his nerves and successfully restored movement to the arm". He spent

---

66 Carver 1978.

the summer recovering in Oxford with his wife.

The story is told as if it was nothing extraordinary, just another British soldier keeping a stiff upper lip! Despite his extensive wounds, he made a remarkable recovery and in October he was graded A by the medical board – fit for any job in his rank. He went on to have a splendid career.

According to the notes that Lord Harding wrote for 'Hana' in 1974, Seddon also restored movement to his right leg. Then "Nov. 1943 appointed to command 8th Corps, a formation allotted to 'Overlord' invasion of Europe – delighted and excited – visited and talked to all units and formations – intent on ensuring lessons learnt for future operations."

War wounds were often multiple and complex, and treatment could take years. In the case of one of Seddon's patients, a Dutch air gunner, Leendert Jonker, we have much circumstantial detail because he told his story to Everard Bakker.[67] As a casualty he was transferred from one hospital to another before he was operated on by Seddon for his nerve injuries; his post-operative treatment continued for years. This is how his saga began:

> 25th October 1943. It looked like any other day so ordinary, but ... 52 crew members of the 320th squadron of the Netherlands Fleet Air Arm had to report early in the morning for a special bombing-mission over enemy territory across the Channel. The target was the airport Lanveoc-Poulmec.
>
> Our Squadron-leader explicitly wanted to make a direct hit and flew a long bombing-run well over 40 sec. to reach his goal. But by doing so we flew directly in the path of heavy ack-ack fire. More or less the same time I saw the bomb drop, an enormous explosion took place. Simultaneously our kite was hit and rolled over on its back, whereupon we started nose-diving while spinning around. Thanks goodness this didn't last long as Jan regained control over the plane. Up till now it's a mystery to me how the wings could have stood up to such a tremendous pressure. This all gave me the strength to regain my composure although severely wounded.

---

67 Bakker 2004.

While in a dream, though it seemed more like a nightmare, I was gazing around and noticed more and more flak bursts of exploding ack-ack shells. In the corner of my eye I observed, high above us, two fighters who were coming towards us and once more alarm took possession of me. Somehow I managed to turn the turret towards the aft-end of the plane, in spite of the fact that I couldn't use my right arm, being badly injured, I tried the firing mechanism and to my unspeakable delight the left machine-gun fired. I felt strangely comforted by this action and my hope to reach our base in Good Old Blighty grew by the second. As the two fighters came nearer I recognised, with a sigh of relief, that they were our own Spitfires. Immediately they took charge of us and accompanied us till we were well out of enemy territory.

Although tormented by appalling pain and loss of blood, I crept out of the turret as I wasn't able to stand up. I looked at my right arm and became dumbfounded, it was nearly severed by the elbow and the underarm was hanging on by a strand of my skin. I also suffered immensely of a severe wound in the thigh of my right leg and of lesser cuts and lacerations on back and legs.

While I laid down there, I somehow succeeded to put on an emergency dressing around my arm or what was left over of it. To accomplish this I had to open a package of emergency first aid kit. Our navigator, Claassen, did his utmost to assist me in my efforts but to no avail. Neither did he succeed in injecting me with morphine to soften my pain. Do not ask me how, but during this spell I noticed that the panzer-windows of the fuselage had disappeared, apparently blown away. Beneath me was an enormous hole on account of having lost our bottom-turret. Above me the blue sky. Through all the holes cold air readily found its way into our plane and probably the cold air acted as an anaesthetic and made me feel numb and drowsy, most presumably it also stopped the flow of blood from my numerous wounds.

Despite the extensive damage, the plane landed successfully near Exeter.

With all the speed they could muster, I was taken to the Royal Devon and Exeter Hospital. The medical staff stood awaiting me. Immediately they cut away all the clothes from my body. As they already had identified my blood-group from my identification-disk, straight away I was given a blood transfusion. I just succeeded to pass-on the address of my wife. Last but not least I remember two doctors bending over me, contemplating to amputate my right arm. My answer to his question if they were allowed to experiment with my arm, was affirmative. Then everything blotted out for me. About nine the same evening I partly awoke out of my narcosis and noticed that my arm was still there. The Canadian orthopaedic surgeon attached to the Hospital paid me daily a visit. He told in full what his plans were if the operation would succeed.
The 2nd of Nov. 1943 became a special day for me. I received two official despatches. The first one informed me that I was awarded the Flying Cross with the following mentioning:

As gunner of a Mitchell-bomber of the 320th Squadron RDNAS of the Dutch Fleet Air Arm stationed in the UK, during an air raid on an enemy airfield near Brest (France) on the 25th Oct. 1943 showed exemplary duty, perseverance, courage and high morality after his plane received a direct hit whereby he himself was severely wounded and with disregard for his own condition and carrying on without pain-killers stayed on his post and even after loss of blood, to control himself and ensuring [sic] the others that nothing was wrong with him, by doing so kept the morale of the crew at highest level.

The 2nd letter from Netherlands Naval H.Q. informed me that I had been promoted to the rank of Sergeant. Obviously this was not to be a dry occasion and a toast with a glass of wine concluded this memorable occasion. The Staff decorated my bed and last but not least flowers and a basket of fruit arrived.

The 5th Nov. 1943. The first plaster cast was being renewed. The medical staff also told me that the operation of my arm had been a great success and didn't have to be amputated. The leading surgeon told me what they had done to save my arm and they showed me the x-rays. At last there was some cause for optimism. Furthermore the surgeon told me that Prof. Seddon of Oxford would be contacted and would undertake the experiment of relaying the nerves in my arm in a different course and connect them up again. But first of all the big wounds had to heal.

On 8 November he was transferred to the RAF hospital at Wroughton, where he had two more operations, mainly skin transplants performed by a New Zealand surgeon, Dr Keto.

The time came when Leendert Jonker was sent to Oxford for a consultation with Seddon, with a view to surgery on the nerves around the damaged elbow.

The second week of January 1944 I was taken by ambulance to the Wingfield Morris Hospital. Arriving there, the driver was told to take me to Ripon Hall, an old castle just outside Oxford. The building and the grounds around it looked like a picture taken out of a fairy-tale book.[68] It was tea time when I arrived and I was introduced to the head-nurse who appeared to be very kind and pleasant. She gave me a short summing-up about Ripon Hall. After that, I was invited to afternoon-tea in the dining hall. It was a real English tea only to be found in England. Later I was introduced to

68 Ripon Hall was built on Boars Hill at the end of the nineteenth century for the President of Trinity College. A tower was added later, making it look like a castle. It had glorious views over Oxford. It had become an Anglican theological college but was requisitioned as a hospital/nursing home. It impressed its patients with features like the library.

the staff and other patients; they all wished me well. I also was introduced to the owner of the castle and his adjutant, both pensioned military men. I was given my own room. The nurses were all voluntary staff assisted by helping hands.

I arrived Tuesday and next day I met Dr. Seddon, the well known neurologist [*sic*], and three of his staff-members. There seemed to be some movement in the arm after removing the plaster-cast. They'd never experienced anything like this. No elbow and yet movement. After examination decision was taken to operate. The nerves in my arm had to be altered and relayed, and then needed connecting up again. The operation was to take place on Saturday-morning at the Wingfield Morris Hospital.

Saturday (20-05-44), the operation date. Prof. Seddon and Miss D. Williams[69] was going to perform the operation. It was a great success, we couldn't have wished for a better result. Prof. Seddon pointed out to me that revalidating would take a long time. It was of the greatest importance to exercise a lot and so regain flexibility of my muscles who had gone rather stiff in the meantime. I promised him I would do my utmost.

In as well outside Ripon Hall I had many friends. We often were invited by very prominent people. Many of them had a position at the University. We heard that many discoveries took place especial on Medical level. Most of the patients underwent voluntary treatment. Prof's, assistants and voluntary part-timers amongst them lots of wives of Doctors and Professors. Anyone of them would be available for 24hrs if necessary just to reach the goal they had set themselves to be of service to the patients. Alas many patients were beyond help, especially where operations were too late due to long waiting times. To perform operations this had to happen within 3 months after the accident to have some chance

---

69 This is probably Dorothy Katherine Williams *née* Elliott of Birmingham, FRCS Eng (1924). Stephanie Brooks recalls her as a small lady. There was also a Miss Shirley Williams; Seddon described her as a clinician. She got a PhD for work in the department on electrical stimulation of paralysed muscles. She left to set up a nerve injuries centre for the RAF.

of success. This on account of the nerves in body and limbs. Students and young doctors were highly interested into the research work of the professor. We, the patients, were often asked to go to university-clinics, all expenses paid. Later we found out that expenses were paid by the interested doctors themselves.

At this time in the university, G Weddell and JZ Young were investigating the degeneration and regeneration of nerve fibres to the skin and muscles after peripheral nerve injuries. Blood flow was important to regeneration. Weddell thought he could judge if a paralysed muscle would regain function from observing the degree of muscle fibrillation of the injured limb. Various machines were being developed: for instance, Bauwers and Ritchie worked from 1941 on a special stimulator that gave alternating current pulses of 50 cycles per second, and these could be measured. Seddon used it during operations to test nerve conduction.

Some doctors thought that even torn off limbs could be affixed again. In my case this was proven. Prof. Seddon and Dr. Zachary [Seddon's assistant after Highet was lost] were of the opinion that nerves could be transplanted. But before this could be achieved, extensive research had to be done. Many makeshift therapies were being tried out special regarding revalidation. Everyday massage, warm bath's and electric shock-therapy. It soon became obvious that, in my case, the doctors were very successful. The "ELBOW" movement and the re-growth of the implanted nerves were going according to plan. Dr. Williams was very proud how things had turned out after the successful operation.

A remarkable incident took place when I visited a theatre in Oxford. During music played on a violin I became increasingly aware of a strong tingling in my arm. It seemed as if I was pricked by thousands of needles. This irritation forced me to leave the theatre.

Of course the weather had great influence on my arm especially by atmospheric pressure. I know now I have to live with this. If stiffening of the muscles take place in my arm it's hellish, but one must fight this continuously and be thankful one is alive and so the remedy is, keep active. Perspiration test amongst others showed that the nerves grew by appr. 1/2 millimetre a day.

The Ripon Hall surroundings were of great beauty, slightly similar to a small place in Holland called Bergen, situated along the North-Sea coast in North Holland. Back to Ripon Hall, woody countryside with many big manors, some farms and last but not least the local pubs. During the war the big houses and manors were filled to the *nock* with all kinds of valuable treasures from all kinds of *musea*.

The hall merged with the church played a great role as a social and cultural centre. We, that's a few patients, were also allowed to take part in this circle. Every Tuesday night card games were being organised. Wednesday-evening was dancing night. Saturday-night there usually was either a film or play-acting. Sunday-morning Church Service and in the evening a forum was formed where all kinds of discussions took place. Social, political and scientific subjects were usually the main items on the menu. Even the local population as well the patients took part in this discussions. Of course the pubs regularly frequented by us for a bite or drink and sometimes for both. During the daytime we were very busy with all kinds of therapy as special attention was given that our damaged limbs etc. would function more or less normal in the future. Even patients were given the opportunity to learn a new trade for times to come. After the invasion in Normandy, the hall was packed with new patients so logically we had to make room for them. Although every 3 months we had to come back for a medical check-up.

Post-operative care and rehabilitation were organised nationally by Brigadier Hugh Cairns, as Director General of Medical Services of the British Army. As a rule, service personnel were not permitted to stay in hospital for more than 180 days.

Chapter 7

Oxford reunion, Don Brooks and the Dutch airman

In Oxford, a few months before operating on the Dutch airman, Seddon opened an interesting parcel sent by Macmillan. It was a gift of Hamilton Bailey's newest text book – not a review copy, though he hoped that Seddon would recommend it to colleagues. Macmillan also offered to see him – if he had made any progress on his book.

CM/MS   17th November, 1943

Dear Professor Seddon,

HAMILTON BAILEY; SURGERY OF MODERN WARFARE
THIRD EDITION. PART1 – 15 s. NET

I know you are very interested in all literature relating to War Surgery.

We have just published Part 1 of this important publication, a presentation copy of which is sent herewith. You will observe that on account of paper restrictions it now appears in its battle dress.

We hope to publish this work in six similar parts. Part II should be ready by the end of this month, Part III in December and Parts IV to VI will appear between January and March 1944.

Your own contribution will appear in a later Part but I thought you would like to have this Part for your own personal use.

If you can recommend it to those interested, we shall esteem this a great favour.

LATEST AND RECENT PUBLICATIONS

ANDERSON. An Introduction to Bacteriological Chemistry.

Second Edition in Preparation. By C. G. ANDERSON, Ph.D.(Birm.), D.Bact.(Lond.), Bacteriological Chemist, Wellcome Physiological Research Laboratories. Crown 8vo, 288 pp. Illustrated with Diagrams. Price, **10s. 6d.** net. Postage, **6d.** (1944.)

The above details apply to the first edition of this book which has been out of print for some time. A Second Edition is in course of preparation and will be published in 1944. The book will be completely revised and brought up to date and some increase may be anticipated in the extent and in the published price.—*Publishers' Note.*

BAILEY. Surgery of Modern Warfare.

Third Edition in Preparation. Edited by HAMILTON BAILEY, F.R.C.S., Surgeon, Royal Northern Hospital, London, etc. *Compiled by Seventy-seven Eminent Contributors from all parts of the world.* Complete in 6 cloth bound parts. Royal medium 8vo, 160 pp. per part, fully illustrated, many in colour. Price, **15s.** net per part. Postage: Inland **6d.** Parts I, II, III, now ready. Parts IV-VI ready shortly. (1944.)

The new Third Edition in preparation is to be published in a series of six parts which will be sold separately. The exact extent and the published prices of the separate parts may vary, but in all probability they will be published at 15s. net per part. The Series will be complete on the publication of Part VI, at the end of which an index will be printed covering the complete work. The reason why the Third Edition is to be published in this form is the urgent need which exists to make available with the least possible delay the latest advances and experience gained in the surgery of modern warfare.—*Publishers' Note.*

BAILEY. Operative Surgery for Nurses.

New Book. In the Press. By HAMILTON BAILEY, F.R.C.S., Surgeon, Royal Northern Hospital, London, etc.

BAILEY. 101 Clinical Demonstrations for Nurses.

New Book. In the Press. By HAMILTON BAILEY, F.R.C.S., Surgeon, Royal Northern Hospital, London, etc.

BIGGART. Pathology of the Nervous System.

By J. HENRY BIGGART, M.D.(Belfast), Professor of Pathology, Queen's University, Belfast. With a Foreword by Professor A. MURRAY DRENNAN, M.D., F.R.C.P.E., University of Edinburgh. Demy 8vo, 350 pp. 204 half-tone illustrations. Price, **15s.** net. Postage, **7d.**

13. Advertisement for Hamilton Bailey's book in patriotic red white and blue, and Publisher's note.

PUBLISHERS' NOTE

Messrs. Livingstone regret that owing to paper shortage it is impossible for them to continue printing their full catalogue of publications.

This list is accordingly confined to the latest new books and new editions and to titles which are still in print and in constant demand.

They will be pleased to answer enquiries about any other works published by them which do not appear in this list.

Further, they wish to explain that the sales of books are now so greatly increased that, together with paper restrictions, it is practically impossible to keep any list of publications up-to-date. An endeavour will be made to meet this circumstance by printing additional lists from time to time as the need arises. Particulars will be given therein of further new titles published and changes in the editions of existing titles.

It should be noted that all the books in this list are strictly net and cannot be procured for less than the published price.

Every effort will be made to have orders despatched the same day as received, provided they are accompanied by a remittance for the net published price, plus postage.

Finally, in the interests of economy in paper, Messrs. Livingstone request that this catalogue, when finished with, be passed on to someone likely to be interested.

During the war, everything was affected by shortages, rationing and austerity. As a result, someone was always collecting something to be re-used. Books were no exception and they were appreciated by soldiers, who often suffered lengthy periods of boredom interspersed by violent bursts of activity. The *Evening Dispatch* of 9 August 1944 featured 'Books for the Forces: General Alexander's Appeal to the Public' asking for suitable books and magazines to be handed in at post offices.

Macmillan's mention of "battle dress" refers to the restrictions imposed on the publishing industry by the Book Production War Economy Agreement. This dictated the size of type to be used, the minimum number of words to the square inch, the weight and quality of paper, and so on. Seddon thanked Macmillan:

> These books are invaluable to us.
> I have been working on the book on Peripheral Nerve Injuries, but progress has been slow because of the immense pressure of work. Recently it has been necessary to operate, sometimes running two tables, on Saturdays, morning and afternoon. It is always a pleasure to talk to you, but so far as the book is concerned there is nothing to discuss at present; I would prefer to wait until I have written a few more chapters.

Twin-table surgery was developed towards the end of the First World War. This system was used where surgeons were under pressure: one patient was anaesthetised while surgery was started on another already anaesthetised.[70] Seddon performed this in partnership with his anaesthetist, with a mastery of timing.

Macmillan wrote again with resigned disappointment:

> I am glad to hear that you find Surgery of Modern Warfare so helpful.
> I note that you have not made the expected progress with your book on Peripheral Nerve Injuries and I do not wish to come through to Oxford unnecessarily. ... If I find I am through in Oxford I shall give you a ring on the telephone in the hope that it may be possible just to

70 Harrison 2004b.

have a word with you but I assure you I shall not trouble you unduly.

There is one point on which I would like your help. Professor Illingworth was anxious to use three illustrations from Mr. Highet's article which appeared in The Lancet. The Lancet has today sent me these blocks and they say we can use them, subject to obtaining permission from you, in the Second Edition of Professor Illingworth's" Textbook of Surgical Treatment." I understand that Professor Illingworth was writing to you direct and all that I am anxious to know is – have we your permission? I enclose a proof of the blocks in question.

The first edition of Illingworth's textbook had been published in 1943 but new methods, particularly of treating burns, meant that a second edition was swiftly commissioned and came out in 1945. It had mainly Scottish contributors and was designed for the Scottish market. The pictures requested by Macmillan were of metal and leather hand splints designed by Highet to support and relax certain muscles. One looked like a knuckle-duster and held the fingers at an angle to the palm. Seddon gave permission to use them.

On 24 January 1944, Seddon explained to Macmillan that there would be more delay to the manuscript

Dear Mr Macmillan,

Thank you very much for Part III of "Surgery of Modern Warfare"; you really are most generous.

In December and during the first week of this month I was getting on splendidly with the book, but during the last seventeen days I have not written a single word. The volume of clinical work coming to us has been suddenly increased by the return of repatriated prisoners of war and I am very much afraid that there will be no spare time at all for some months to come. Furthermore, my Malta affairs are boiling up again.

I see no hope whatever of completing this work by the end of February and circumstances are such that I cannot even name a later finishing date. I shall be grateful if you will explain this to Mr. Walker and assure that the delay is due to circumstances over which I have no control.

The many released prisoners of war brought not only more cases but also fresh problems. One of those referred to Seddon thought he had been well treated in a German hospital, but his injuries had left him with a limp arm. Seddon judged it was now probably too late for an operation to repair the nerves to be effective.

In 1944 Seddon was at last re-united with his family. They sailed into Liverpool on board the troopship *Mauretania* – in peace-time the fast Cunard liner – and travelled by train to Oxford. The meeting at the station was a tender moment in more than one sense because he had a large swelling on his chin from a bee sting. The government encouraged bee-keeping because of the contribution honey made to the national diet, but Seddon had to give it up because of his hypersensitivity to stings. When Mary and the children moved back to Oxford, they and Granny found it difficult to live together harmoniously.

Mary had an excellent arts degree from Bryn Mawr, the prestigious college in Pennsylvania, but she never pursued any career beyond housewife and mother. In later years, when her husband and children had achieved great things, they found it very difficult to understand Mary's lack of motivation or ambition. She did arrange programmes of visits and entertainment for the wives of visiting academics and surgeons. Apart from that, she was probably busy enough caring for the family and enjoying a social life with friends from academic families.

The Seddon family house, 66 Old Road (Fig 2), was right opposite the hospital and almost next door to Professor Girdlestone's home. Many of the patients in the Wingfield-Morris were children, and young James in particular found it most distressing at night to hear them crying either because they were in pain or just because of the strange surroundings. Seddon himself was very aware of this. Donal Brooks, one of his junior surgeons at the time, recalls how

Jim's kindness and gentleness and great sense of fun gave much needed reassurance to parent and child alike. Children loved him, and he was never so happy as when amongst his 'chicks'.

On coming home from work Jim would take a bath before anything else, to prevent spreading infection to his own children. They were sent to Headington High, a girls' school that also admitted a few boys to its most junior part. Both children were very clever, but Sally was ill-prepared for an old-fashioned English school after so much time in America and was a bit of a tom-boy. James was teased for his American accent and was relieved when he moved to the Dragon School in 1947. Sally remembers her father had a real love and gift of gardening:

> The house was pleasant enough, but with not a lot of character, but it was the garden that was a real joy. With allotments in the distance at the back of a large garden and nobody overlooking us, it had the feel of a true country garden and the fruit was outstanding. There were cherries, plums, quinces as well as masses of apples to harvest. He [her father] rigged up a pulley from the loft and, with the help of lots of small Dragons from James's school, the apples were hauled up to the loft in baskets and stored. He made the most amazing rock garden out of a huge hole in the ground some fifty feet long which was famous throughout Oxford, and quite lovely in May. He also grew dahlias.

Family holidays were full of fun and some unexpected adventures. Once, on holiday by the sea, they called to see a friend who had a pet donkey. The poor animal had torn an eyelid on a nail in its shed. Could the surgeon please repair it? Sally was sent off to the nearby chemist to procure ether or chloroform. The suspicious pharmacist asked how much? – "Enough to anaesthetise a donkey" was the answer. Jim held a cloth soaked in the stuff to the donkey's nose. The donkey immediately took off around the field while Jim clung on, with one arm round its neck and the other holding the improvised Schimmelbush mask. Gradually the anaesthetic took effect and the beast subsided onto the grass, but unfortunately on to the wrong side. They rolled it over and son James was told to sit on it. This he did, but with his fists in his eyes so he should not have to see the operation. Jim sewed up the eyelid with darning needle and thread, and the donkey made a full recovery. However, someone had seen the capers in the field and reported to the RSPCA that they had seen a donkey being cruelly treated. Jim had some explaining to do. This became a story that Donal Brooks loved to tell.

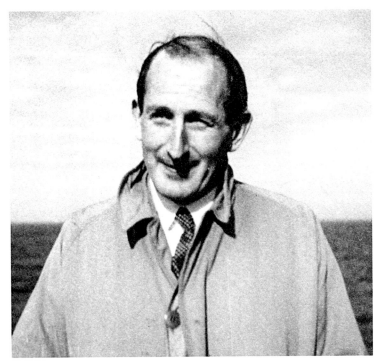

14. Jim on holiday

It was while Seddon was away in Malta that Girdlestone, the previous Professor of Orthopaedics, interviewed Donal Brooks, a graduate of Trinity College, Dublin. He had come over from Ireland, where orthopaedics was not recognised as a separate branch of surgery at that time. As a child he had had surgery that left him with a slight limp, so he was unfit for active service during the war. Brooks was a day late for interview and his papers had been lost by officials, but Seddon's secretary just happened to know a schoolfriend's father who was the man to put things right. Two other candidates had already been interviewed, but fortunately Girdlestone was prepared to wait to see Brooks, who was selected for the post.

Don's appointment to the peripheral nerve injury unit in 1944 was the beginning of a successful partnership with Jim Seddon that would last many years. This is how Don remembers it:

I came to Oxford in 1944 when the hospital still housed many wounded Servicemen, and the Peripheral Nerve Injury Unit was a flourishing concern. The first and overwhelming impression of H.J.S. was of a man who was very precise and accurate in recording his own observations, and who expected his juniors to be the same, always insisting that their observations should be written down at the time. His strict regard for accuracy and intellectual honesty made him a welcome collaborator with scientists in other departments of the university, in particular J. Z. Young and Peter Medawar in the Department of Zoology. It was these links, and others, that enabled him to establish a scientific basis for the clinical research that he was undertaking on peripheral nerve injuries. There is no doubt that it was this background, together with his capacity for ensuring a high quality of note taking and recording, that established the international reputation of the Oxford Peripheral Nerve Injury Centre – one of the five set up by the Medical Research Council in Britain.

Because he expected those around him to have his own standards of honesty and precision, he was always prepared to delegate a good deal of responsibility, and his delight knew no bounds when a member of the team showed sufficient initiative to establish a reputation in some aspect of the joint work. It is hardly surprising that he gathered round him a team of men and women who gladly and unsparingly gave of their best to him.[71]

Backing up the team there were the secretaries for the clinical and research units. Of the four lively research secretaries, there was one who had been seconded from Ripon Hall aged only 15; she became Seddon's personal secretary when his existing secretary joined up. Stephanie had been trained at an elite secretarial college, Woodlees, near Blenheim, and might have become secretary to an MP but, before that could happen, because all 16-year-olds had to take a job, she found herself working in a hospital. She joined the secretaries in the research department. Dr Zachary was very helpful in explaining medical terms, but the secretaries had to puzzle out a shorthand way of writing words like axontmesis.

Stephanie also had to look after the punched cards that held data on each patient in the research projects. Punched cards were a simple but effective way of holding information so it could be sorted into groups. Around the edge of each card were holes through which a rod such as a knitting needle could be thrust and groups of cards lifted out. If the hole extended to the edge of the card, then the needle would fail to lift it out. If you punched open the hole in the A5 position, say, for all patients aged between 20 and 30, then a needle poked through that hole would leave all those cards behind. But beware any clumsy move or they would all go flying, as Stephanie learnt.

Work was hard, but there was time for amateur theatricals – such as the annual hospital pantomime, in which the secretaries took leading parts – and dances. Seddon thought he should learn to dance the tango so one of the secretaries tried to teach him. However, though musical, he did not quite grasp the the essential exuberance of the moves; it was more of a mathematical exercise. At least he tried!

He was so focused on his work that he lacked insight into much else that was going on. He was puzzled to find Donal (or Don,

---

71 Brooks 1978.

as he was better known) hanging about so often outside his office. The reason was a mystery to Jim until it became clear that Don had fallen in love with Stephanie, the girl whose initiative and contacts had got him to his interview in the first place. They had a grand wedding at Holy Trinity, Brompton Road in London, and invited many from the hospital to the reception at the Hyde Park Hotel. Afterwards Stephanie had to give up work and Seddon had to find a new secretary.

He probably also had to plan what books his students would need in the next academic year. Basil Blackwell, the bookseller and publisher, had written to Veale, the registrar of the university, to say that there was a desperate shortage of books and he needed to know what to order for the next intake of students. Then on 26 January 1944 there was yet another letter from Macmillan, replying to Jim's explanation of the delay to his own book.

> My heart gave a flutter when I noticed a letter from you. I thought it would be inviting me down to discuss the Pros. and Cons. of your book.
>
> I fully sympathise with the views you have expressed and the present time is not the best for doing a serious work like writing a Textbook. Sometimes, however, the best results are obtained while under pressure and it has been true throughout all history that those with the heaviest burdens are always the most fruitful and I am hoping against hope that one day I will receive this summons to Oxford.
>
> If I am in the vicinity, of course, I will certainly let you know as I always enjoy my conversations with you. Therefore, do your very utmost but at the same time do not feel under undue bondage as far as our firm is concerned.
>
> Your last paragraph made me realise that I have failed in my duty. I thought I had reported to you earlier that our Mr. Walker died suddenly on August 8th last. His death was most unexpected and I am afraid it has involved me in quite a lot of extra responsibility. We are negotiating with the Trustees and they have asked Mr.

Scott and myself to be responsible for carrying on the publishing firm of E. & S. Livingstone. I hope to be in a position soon to give you exact information about this change which I feel sure you will be interested in.

Macmillan continued to send books to Seddon, who continued to be grateful:

23rd June, 1944

Dear Mr. Macmillan,

Thank you for your continued generosity; I agree Part VI is really first-rate though, as yet, I have only had time to look through it quickly.

No, there is no prospect of my completing the book on nerve injuries within the near future. This work of ours becomes more and more time-consuming and had I known what would be happening I should never have given any kind of undertaking. Nevertheless, the preparation of the book is continuing and one day it will be finished.

He might not be finding time for his book but he did find time to write an article for *The Practitioner* on 'The early management of peripheral nerve injuries'.[72] It had such an effect on one young man in Leeds, who found it "so different, so exciting", that he networked his way to Oxford to ask Seddon if he could work for him. He was just one of many inspired by Seddon to take up orthopaedics. There was no vacancy, but Seddon found a post for him in the Radcliffe with Jim Scott – and that was how Max Harrison began the career of orthopaedic surgeon. On D Day, Wing-Commander Jim Scott was stationed at the Wingfield-Morris chiefly to organise reception into three of the wards of those casualties from the landings in France with unusually severe injuries.

In France, another young man had started on a surgical career. He had been taken prisoner early in the hostilities and treated French and German soldiers. Released to pursue his training in Lyon, he cycled to join resistance fighters in the fastness of the Ardèche. His name was Albert Trillat and after the war he got to know Seddon

---

72 Seddon 1944.

and his family. As a senior orthopaedic surgeon in Lyon he introduced the 'no touch' methods he had learnt in England: sterile instruments were carefully laid out on a towel and the surgeon and staff
were permitted to touch only the handles. This method, which Sir
William Arbuthnot Lane (1856–1943) introduced and taught to his
disciples until his retirement in 1920, prevented micro-contamination
and reduced infection of a wound. Lane had specially designed
instruments with long handles.[73]

At the Wingfield-Morris extra help arrived when a Danish
orthopaedic surgeon, Dr John Agerholm-Christensen, joined the
team, having managed to escape from imprisonment by the SS. At
the same time, other staff were leaving to continue their careers
elsewhere, partly because the number of casualties sent to the unit
for nerve repairs was decreasing. Between 1944 and 1945 the number
of patients attending Ripon Hall dropped by about a fifth, to an
average of 55 a day receiving treatment there. Ripon Hall closed at
the end of 1946.

At its wartime peak, the number of patients at the
Wingfield-Morris had more than doubled and the workshops must
have been very busy making prostheses. In 1944 the Minister of
Pensions formed a committee to consider the design, development
and use of artificial limbs and appliances; Seddon was among its
members.

In the final days of the European war, one of the patients
arriving at St Hugh's – the women's college which had been turned
into a military hospital for head wounds – was a young man with multiple injuries who saw penicillin being used to great effect on the
medical wards there. When the young man was transferred to
Seddon's unit at the Wingfield-Morris for surgery on his leg, the
professor was away in Mauritius, so his first assistant undertook the
operation.

Robert Bransby Zachary had graduated first in pharmacy in
1935 and then in medicine in 1940 at Leeds. He had been
recommended by Max Harrison to come to Oxford. The wounded
soldier said "[Zachary] a very nice hunchback allowed me to watch
over my shoulder while he operated on the nerve behind my knee,
with very fair success on what had been complete footdrop". The

---

73 Clarke 1966.

frayed torn nerve was trimmed and re-united, but was now shorter, so the leg was set at an angle and encased in a reinforced plaster. Over the following weeks this was adjusted, using a locally made gadget.

Only two months later the young man was a medical student at Worcester College, where his tutor was Bill Holmes, who worked with JZ Young on nerve repair. Bill gave him a souvenir of his operation – a small piece of his nerve. At this time Holmes was writing a paper with Seddon about the blood supply to a cut nerve.[74] At the college, this patient also met Seddon and was able to tell him that he was now fit enough to ski in the Alps. Later Seddon demonstrated him as a model of successful peripheral nerve injury repair at a meeting of the Royal Society of Medicine.

Physiotherapists had an important place in treatment of orthopaedic patients. On 29 September Seddon was invited to address their Congress. He spoke about 'The treatment of lower motor neuron lesions'. [75]

One of the physical therapies used to prevent muscle atrophy until the nerve repair was effective was called galvanic stimulation. Flight Lieutenant ECS Jackson, RAFVR, and Seddon published an item on this therapy.[76] Interstitial fibrosis was "a constant feature of denervation atrophy of muscles without a motor nerve supply". Repeated electric stimulation of the muscle was tried to counter this atrophy – and believed to be beneficial. Treatment was given six days a week. Early experimentation was done with animals, but good results were later found not so common in humans. "Although galvanism has several disadvantages – the discomfort it causes being one of the most important – it is still the only type of stimulus of long duration generally available, and it was for this reason that it was used in the investigation to be tried". Would fibrillation tire the muscle out and make matters worse? Some were critical of this therapy, considering the only thing that mattered was good surgery – that is, good apposition of the axons.[77]

One of the problems of nerve surgery was to get the nerve fibres to grow down the Schwann tubes without encountering a block or going astray, and then to make satisfactory connections.

---

74 Seddon and Holmes 1945.
75 Seddon 1945c.
76 Jackson and Seddon 1945.
77 Abercrombie 1945.

Ruth Bowden used electromycography to assess the denervation and re-inervation in human voluntary muscle.[78] "The finding of both fibrillation and motor-unit potentials indicates a partial or recovering degenerative lesion of the lower motor neurone".[79] Thus electromycography was used to assess nerve function.

Even when treatment was successful, it could be difficult to provide aftercare. For instance, the final phase of the Dutch air gunner's treatment could only take place after his employer had assigned him to a different post.

> In July 1944 I was given leave and travelled to Holyhead where my wife lived. First I had to report aboard Hr. Ms. Depotship "Medusa", formerly a minelayer. Medically they could not treat me in Holyhead. Prof. Seddon suggested I put in for a transfer, to be stationed in London. The professor would personally be able to attend me. So the Dutch Navy had to create a position for me. After consultation with the Naval Officer in charge of the Personnel Dept. I was put in charge of the project "Watertransport" which meant I had to take care of Dutch Naval personnel, their wives and children who were repatriated to Holland, and looking after their personal belongings.
>
> For further medical treatment I had to attend a R.A.F. clinic in Regents Park. From September 1944 up to and including May 1947 I have been in medical care. So within 11 months after my disastrous flying mission I resumed active service in the Dutch Naval Force.

Being such an interesting and successful case, Leendert Jonker had some interesting encounters:

> Soon after one of my daily visits to the clinic I was to meet highly placed functionaries. Sir Winston Churchill was one of them. He was being troubled by a painful back. We rather got on well and this resulted in an

---

78 Bowden 1945.
79 Weddell, Feinstein and Pattle 1943.

invitation to attend a session of Parliament. I even was presented with two of his famous cigars. As well ministers and high ranking officers, amongst them Chief of Staff of the R.A.F., underwent therapeutic treatment.

But these visits were just a prologue of what was going to be one of my greatest and most memorable encounter of all. One morning, during treatment, the Doctor and a courier from Buckingham Palace entered the massage-room. This Royal Messenger introduced himself and revealed to me that he had to pass on a request from His Majesty King George the Sixth. The Royal Request was phrased as follows: His Majesties King George and Queen Elizabeth with both the Royal Highnesses Elizabeth and Margaret intended to pay a visit to the R.A.F. clinic and H.M. the King would appreciate it very much if Sergeant L. Jonker would also be present that particular day. The Royal visit would take place the week after. Miss Williams my physiotherapist as well as myself were overcome with delight and looking forward to this memorable occasion. I pledged myself by ensuring the Courier that I would not fail to be present. It seemed that only one officer of the Dutch Navy Air Arm was informed of this Royal Visit.

During the visit I felt completely relaxed. Miss Williams continued her normal treatment as usual. His Majesty the King was completely informed about my military career in the Marine Corps and the Dutch Fleet Air Arm. His Majesty also asked questions about medical treatment in three hospitals and how they managed to save my arm. The doctor who accompanied the Royal Family pointed out to the king how important this was for the medical world to achieve this success. I have no exact recollection of the time how long the Royal visit lasted, but I believe longer than 35 minutes. The parting of this memorable visit was also something to be remembered, full of warmth and understanding.

I paid a visit to the Wingfield Morris Hosp. in Sept

1947; the main reason, I was still being bothered by painful nerves attacks in the stomach-region. Prof. Seddon told me that the symptoms I mentioned plus troubled vocal chords and occasionally nightmares was the most common complaint of flying personnel who participated in nightly operations also those who had been under great strain. These complaints reveal themselves approximately 6 months after a long period of rest. He warned me strongly not to take painkillers, alcohol and any other sedative. He advised me to keep myself bodily as well as mentally fit. To keep one goal in life based on the future making good use of knowledge and experience gained during life. There's no better healing remedy according to him. At long last I bade farewell to the Professor, doctors and the entire nursing staff. At last, the injuries and the experimental treatment I received contributed a step forwards in the medical world.

Chapter 8

Peace – but not in Oxford

Charles Macmillan and Alfred J Scott were made joint Managing Directors of E & S Livingstone, but this partnership was destined to be short-lived, as Macmillan explained to Seddon on 22 January 1945:

> Dear Professor Seddon,
>
> <u>BONE GRAFTING IN THE TREATMENT OF FRACTURES 25s. NET.</u>
>
> We have just published this Monograph by Mr. J. R. Armstrong and I thought you would be more than interested in it. Therefore I have great pleasure in sending you a presentation copy.
>
> After perusal I hope you will be able to bring it to the attention of your colleagues and friends and if you can use your influence to help us in introducing this book I will feel most grateful for any help you can give us in this direction.
>
> I have not bothered you about your own book on Peripheral Nerve Injuries. There have been a series of catastrophes here. We had just got the Company going nicely when most unexpectedly my co-Director, Mr Alfred James Scott, died suddenly on 5th October last. Then at the end of October a disastrous fire occurred at one of our printing factories and 90% of all the coloured illustrations in our publications were completely destroyed.
>
> These two incidents involved me in a considerable amount of extra work and I have not been able to follow up past connections.
>
> I hope, however, that one day soon you will be in a position to give my firm the honour of producing something from your pen.

I trust you keep well despite the tremendous strain the war years must have laid on you.
With Kind Regards,
I am,
Yours sincerely,
E. & S. LIVINGSTONE, LTD.
Charles Macmillan
MANAGING DIRECTOR.

Seddon was worried about his health and he was grateful for Macmillan's concern. The heavy work load during the war and difficult medico-political affairs had stretched Seddon to the limit of his strength.

Germany surrendered on 6 May. Victory in Europe was celebrated as VE Day on the 8th. Japan surrendered a few months later. Britain was impoverished and people were exhausted by the war effort, but with the war ended there was optimism for a brighter future. Now the health of the nation needed some attention.

Levels of tuberculosis (TB) had risen, but the disease was now potentially curable with chemotherapy. The first effective antibiotic for the disease was streptomycin, developed at the Mayo Clinic in Minnesota from a British cultured source. Physicians found that the TB bacillus developed resistance to the antibiotic and patients relapsed. Then a physician working in Edinburgh, John Crofton (knighted in 1977), used the brilliant strategy of triple therapy by adding two other agents, para-amino-salicylic acid (PAS) and isoniazid. From 1954 this drug regime, combined with energetic efforts to identify cases in the population, almost wiped out TB in Britain. A vaccine for TB was developed in France by Calmette and Guerin before the war but not used widely in Britain until 1945. Eventually there would also be a vaccine against polio.

Although the Beveridge report had been published in December 1942, there was much planning and argument before the National Health Service was established. Among the obstacles was the resistance of the medical profession, revealed in August 1944 in a survey of doctors' views by the British Institute of Public Opinion. A new era in the history of medicine was being born, and change in the practice of medicine was inevitable.

Medical textbooks were needed for teaching all the new discoveries of modern medicine to the post-war generation of medical students and postgraduates, so there was potential for E & S Livingstone to grow. Macmillan sent Seddon a book by Ian Smillie, who later became Professor of Orthopaedics at the University of St Andrews.

27th March, 1946.

Dear Mr Macmillan,

It really is most kind of you to send me a copy of Mr. Smillie's book; I know something of his work and I have a great admiration for him.

The book on nerve injuries is still making no progress at all. This, I can honestly say is not my fault, since conditions here are still very far from normal.

So I am in the unhappy position of wanting to see you just because it would be so pleasant to meet again – and yet dreading your visit because of the expression of gentle reproach which I am sure your face would betray.

My kindest regards to you

One nurse's memories were of enjoying enormously the chance to see Professor Seddon do exploration and suture of numerous nerve injuries. She observed that Professor Seddon asked for a glass of milk between cases and the nurses wondered if he had an ulcer, as that was the recommended diet for the condition at that time, though it was later found to be more likely to irritate the stomach.[80] Seddon was indeed not well, as he explained to his employer at the Faculty of Medicine.

Dear Margoliouth,

On the advice of Dr Cooke I am going away for six weeks. There is nothing seriously wrong but for some time past I have not been doing my work properly. I

---

80 Reminiscences of the Wingfield Morris Hospital (Jay Stookes) Centre for Oxfordshire Studies.

think I made the mistake of not taking proper holidays but now that something like normal conditions are returning I hope to avoid that error in future. Would you be good enough to explain the circumstances to such of the University as should be notified.[81]

A summer meeting of the RSM Orthopaedic Section was usually held outside London and in mid-June of 1946 it came to the Wingfield-Morris Hospital. The short papers given included one by Seddon on 'Peripheral nerve grafting operations' and also a cinematograph film and talk by him on 'Muscle transplantation: portion of the pectoris major muscle to paralysed biceps'. This was followed by tea in the Nuffield block.[82]

It was early the next year before Macmillan wrote to Seddon again, on 17 January 1947:

I am coming to London next week for a Meeting of the Medical Group of the Publishers Association.

I would like to come through to Oxford on Thursday, 23rd instant, primarily to see you and to have a chat with you about Peripheral Nerve Injuries. Do not be alarmed, I am not coming to place some fresh obligation on your shoulders, but rather to have a friendly discussion!

I thought I would try to contact Dr. Trueta at the same time but it might not be suitable for either you or Dr. Trueta to see me on this particular day ...

At the same time, I would very much like to meet you again and I sincerely hope that it will be possible for you to grant me an interview.

With Kind Regards

Trueta was now Technical Adviser to the Emergency Medical Service and an Acting Surgeon at the Wingfield-Morris Hospital. His treatment methods of severe injuries had allowed wounds to heal more quickly than before and the next stage

---

81 Letter of 24 April 1946, FA6/15/2. Herschel Maurice Margoliouth (1887–1959), poet and literary historian, was Secretary of Faculties for the University of Oxford.
82 Royal Society of Medicine Archives. Section on Orthopaedics.

operation on damaged nerves could proceed. After the war Trueta remained in Oxford and his research focused on the effects of blood loss on kidney function. Macmillan probably did not try to recruit him as an author as Trueta already had a publisher, but he would have found his opinions useful. Trueta had published work in Spain before the war and in 1943 his work *The Principles and Practice of War Surgery with Special Reference to the Biological Method of Treatment of Wounds* was published by Hamish Hamilton Medical together with William Heinemann Medical.[83] These were just two of the many medical publishers with whom E & S Livingstone were in competition.

The Spirit of Catalonia – Trueta's account of the Spanish Civil War[84] – had been published in 1946 and Trueta loved talking about his life. Macmillan probably enjoyed his many stories too for, as Seddon remarked, "It was always a pleasure to see his fine figure and handsome, vivacious face, and to listen to him, even though he never quite understood that going at top speed in a foreign tongue was not exactly the same as fluency".[85] Even years later Seddon could not resist a waspish sting about the rival to whom he lost the Oxford chair.

After their meeting Macmillan wrote to Seddon:

It was a real joy to meet you again after so many years and to have the friendly talk together.

I am sure one day I will be getting your book on "Injuries to the Peripheral Nerves" and you know if at any time I can be of service to you in the production of your work, you need not hesitate to let me know.

I also hope I shall hear from Dr. Trueta and get his views about the proposed book on "Local Analgesia."

With Kind Regards

The first meeting of the International Society of Orthopaedic Surgery since the war took place in Brussels in October 1947. Seddon was there and showed a film of joint movements of foot, knee and upper limbs. This was the cineradiography done with Dr AE Barclay that had been shown as preliminary work to the

---

83 Trueta 1943.
84 Trueta 1946.
85 Seddon 1977.

British Orthopaedic Association. It was also shown at the American Academy of Orthopaedic Surgeons, where it was awarded the Certificate of Merit.[86]

Seddon was invited to America to give the Charles Mayo Memorial Lecture. He chose as his subject 'Use of autogenous grafts for the repair of large gaps in peripheral nerves'.[87] This invitation may have came about because of his contacts during the war with Loyal Davis, who after the war became professor and chairman of the Department of Surgery at the Northwestern University Medical School in Chicago, Illinois. It was an irresistible invitation. Jim and Mary both wanted to visit America again, so they made arrangements for the children to board for a term. While in the USA, he also read a paper to the American Medical Association.

In Oxford, Seddon's department continued to attract European doctors eager to learn his methods. Yet, despite his high profile, his salary was considerably less than that of the other Nuffield professors. This was an issue that had rumbled on through the war years. It seems the Nuffield Committee for the Advancement of Medicine were aware of this anomaly because on 11 November 1942 they wrote to ask the Hebdomadal Council of the university whether they would raise their contribution to Seddon's salary from £600 to £800. The committee's letter explained that Seddon did not do private work but did have to "attend some paying patients in the Wingfield-Morris Hospital".[88]

On 18 June 1943, Seddon consulted Douglas Veale, the university registrar, about how to go about obtaining a rise in salary:

> I feel especially hesitant about making a fuss. But my circumstances are quite definitely Micawberish and I am compelled to do something. Who is there who would be willing to bother himself about this? The Master of Balliol is the only person I can think of, but I don't know his mind sufficiently well to approach him.

---

86 Seddon 1947a.
87 Seddon 1947b, 1947c.
88 The reports and correspondence quoted in this chapter are all in the Central and Faculty archives and the Nuffield Medical Benefaction in the Bodleian Library at the University of Oxford.

As on so many occasions I shall value your advice; it is always so sound.

    Yours ever
        Herbert Seddon.

The question of private practice complicated the problem. Seddon's appointment did not permit him to keep earnings from private patients; instead the fees, charged in guineas, were paid into the University Chest for the Nuffield Committee. However, he received an annual payment of £600 in lieu.

The next year Girdlestone wrote a lengthy memorandum, dated 10 October 1944. In it he asked that the whole question of university physicians and private patients should be made more explicit. He thought that the Professor of Orthopaedics and Clinical Director of the Wingfield-Morris should get the same salary as other Nuffield professors, namely £2,500. In his opinion the professor should not "engage in private practice" in the sense of becoming "responsible for the care of private patients … He should be able to see them but be relieved of the responsibility for their care". Girdlestone also asked for "a square deal for honorary staff".

It seems the clever new professor was attracting patients in a way that made other surgeons jealous. Girdlestone considered the case of Professor Seddon different from that of Professor Cairns who, Girdlestone felt, could see private patients because his skills were "unique in Oxford". Girdlestone also believed that, even if Seddon was the person to do an operation, nonetheless the honorary surgeon whose patient was being operated on had to be present and continue the care.

When Girdlestone had resigned in 1939 as professor and Clinical Director, to make way for a younger man, Seddon had inherited both posts. In 1946 Mr Jalks, chairman of the Executive Committee of the Wingfield-Morris Hospital, wrote to HM Margoliouth at the Faculty of Medicine:

> I cannot understand why the executive committee ever
> agreed to the present arrangement, under which it is
> liable to have dumped upon it a Clinical Director

appointed to another office, and in virtue of his qualifications for that office (the Professor of Orthopaedic Surgery), by a Board of Electors on which the Hospital is entirely unrepresented. There must be surely some way of dealing with this anomaly, other than by the simple method of cutting the Gordian knot by the Hospital deciding in future to appoint its own Clinical Director, and divorce that office from that of the Professor.

I do not feel that would be satisfactory to either side, but I suppose it might be necessary.

The reply was that the Electors could not be changed, but it was possible for Lord Nuffield to stand aside. The row was a typical Oxford 'town and gown' dispute.

With the introduction of the National Health Service less than a year away, Seddon wrote to the Nuffield Committee on 15 February 1947. He had fewer patients now from the armed services, so money paid by the Ministry of Health for them was drying up. He found it necessary to see private patients to supplement his income. He also grumbled that he had too much administrative work – for clinics at the Radcliffe and hospitals in Aylesbury, Windsor, Newbury, Banbury, Maidenhead and twelve other places. He also had administrative duties in the Wingfield-Morris Hospital and meetings of the Executive Committee. All this left him with no time for research. He wanted a salary of £2,500, like other professors, and not to have to do private work.

The Nuffield Committee replied on 10 March 1947 that they thought it should be a £2,000 salary plus £500 for not keeping private patient fees. The professorship should be severed from the Clinical Director post at the Wingfield-Morris. Seddon wrote to Sir Robert McCarrison, vice-chairman at the Wingfield-Morris Hospital, that "I think this is excellent".

Seddon had become adept at juggling sources of funding for his staff in the Nuffield Unit, using sources in the university, the University Grants Committee, the Nuffield Committee and the Nuffield Dominions Trust, which as its name suggests funded doctors from the Commonwealth or colonies. There were sometimes hiccoughs, as when Zachary did not receive pay for six months while his funding was being transferred from the university to the University Grants Committee.

With the coming of the National Health Service, it was expected that the Wingfield-Morris would become a regional hospital, not a teaching hospital, although Seddon had made a case some years before to the Board of the Faculty of Medicine (of which he was a member) for it to become a university hospital, a proposal "appreciated" by the Faculty board. The university registrar, Veale, had grasped the politics of the situation at that time and wrote to the Vice Chancellor on 17 October 1942 that "I think there is more in this question than meets the eye. The Regional Hospital Council is making a strong bid to get control of the Hospital Services throughout the region." He did not think they would value research and teaching highly. As a result the Medical Advisory Committee recommended closer ties between the Wingfield-Morris Hospital and the university.

The Report of the Committee on the future of the medical school contained a section by Seddon.

In almost all medical schools the chief, in some the only, defect is the abandonment in the wards of the lessons learned in the preclinical departments and even of the habits of thought that inform the scientific pursuits of the early years. Yet when the postgraduate stage is reached, no progress, except in diagnostic acumen and technical proficiency, is possible without constant reference to the basic sciences. We are agreed that our aim is the scientific advancement of medicine. We could, therefore, plan a school for teaching medicine in such a way that clinical work is a natural continuation of all that has gone before. ... That there are scientifically-minded young clinicians in every school is common knowledge, but they exist in virtue of their innate tendencies rather than because their development has been encouraged. And there is little chance of their discovering them and ensuring that they are placed in surroundings where their talents can be put to best use. At least one school in the country should devote itself to training "scientific doctors", and perhaps this is to be one of the contributions to British medicine. From this it follows that the clinical school should be small and, above all, selective.

The report suggested 20 to 25 clinical students. The subjects taught in the clinical school would be "the usual" for final BM, BCh: medicine, surgery, midwifery, special and clinical pathology, forensic medicine and public health. They would include practical experience and tutorials. The committee thought that, though the professors did not want to be taken from their research, they should spend some time teaching undergraduates.

The neurosurgeon Professor Hugh Cairns is quoted in the report:

> One of the main causes for the success of the expanded medical school has been the association of the scientific departments and the new clinical departments in planned research, and the work has received great impetus from the wartime urge of the scientific departments to make practical contributions to the war effort. Among many recent activities may be instanced (1) zoologists, anatomists and surgeons working together on problems of regeneration of peripheral nerves (2) physiologists and experimental psychologist collaborating with neurosurgeons on the subject of brain damage.

After the war the hope was that this would continue. Professor Peters made the point that variety, not nationwide standardisation, was needed. At the end of May 1945, Professor Florey complained about the interminable meetings on the future of the medical school!

In 1946 ML Jalks wrote, as chairman of the Executive Committee of the Wingfield-Morris Hospital, that they supported the status of a teaching hospital within the Medical School of the university for their hospital. In April 1947 the clinics were divided into regional and professorial. The Professorial Unit should have 58 beds, 46 in the hospital (including four in private wards) and 12 in the Churchill Hospital. The 46 represented one quarter of the beds available, other surgeons having the remainder. The Professorial Unit was to be served solely by the professor and his staff. All the facilities should be shared by arrangement.

There was then a row about bed numbers, and the Nuffield Committee took Seddon's side that he needed 58 beds and that it would be embarrassing for him having frequently to seek leave for access to a patient for which his colleague was responsible. Accounts in September 1947 showed bed costs of £800 for patients outside the area but of special interest to Seddon.

His post as Clinical Director of the Wingfield-Morris Hospital was abolished that year; he continued in post as Nuffield professor. It seems clear that the complexity and uncertainty of the situation, along with the number of individuals and bodies concerned, gave scope for political and personal rivalries to complicate even further the transition to new arrangements. Seddon sought and found a way out.

24th May 1948

Dear Turpin

I have accepted an invitation to become Director of Studies at the Institute of Orthopaedics in the University of London and Clinical Director of the Royal National Orthopaedic Hospital. …

I have been increasingly uneasy about the relationship between the Department of Orthopaedic Surgery and the Wingfield Morris Hospital, so much so that I question the possibility of the survival of the Department at any rate under my direction.

A story in circulation shows just how bad relations between Girdlestone and Seddon had become. The former enjoyed a game of golf and, when he teed up, he would imagine the ball to be Seddon's head and then take a good swing at it with a wood. Perhaps Seddon had similar thoughts when dead-heading the flowers in his garden.

In the same letter, Seddon added that he needed to move to London on 1 July 1948 if possible. The Nerve Injuries Unit would be transferred to London; Don Brooks would continue to work with it and his secretary Miss Palmer would also move. However, the situation of Dr Sanders, Mr Mackenzie, Miss Macdonald and Miss Moyle, the junior secretary, would have to be considered.

> In conclusion I feel bound to record my appreciation of the constant encouragement given to me by my friends who make up the Nuffield Committee, during the years when I have been endeavouring to build up what was the first university department of orthopaedic surgery in the country.

His resignation was accepted as from 30 June 1948.

He packed up and departed, taking various bits of equipment with him; as a result, there was some petty correspondence about ownership. On 5 July, when he was sailing on the RMS Queen Mary, he wrote:

> My Dear Ellis
> You obviously did not enjoy telephoning me, in the night before I left, about the matter of the Wingfield equipment. I realise you were trying to scare me from being sent to a sort of academic Ellis Islands, and the least I owe you is a letter. This is not a defence: none is needed. It is simply an explanation.'

As ever, he is systematic:

> There are two things to be considered: what I have done, and the manner in which I did it.

He says that his records show how slender were the resources of the department, and that he became an accomplished scrounger as a result:

I think now that I can get staffing grants out of anybody, though it is always hard work.

Also he says that money paid by the Ministry of Health into his research fund was intended to cover equipment, though some of it was used for salaries:

> The nerve injuries unit, especially during the Ripon Hall days, was like elsewhere, self contained; and when the Ministry of Health agreed, as it did instantly, that it should be transferred to London it was obvious that move had to be a complete one. What is more there was an element of urgency. Because the MRC Report is supposed to be more or less complete by the end of the year (I am Chairman of the Nerve Injuries Committee) we must bring the follow up work completely up to date within the next few months.
>
> Zachary returns in September to work full time till the end of the year.[89] ... If anything I have erred on the side of leaving behind certain articles that might quite properly be regarded as M of H equipment. ...
>
> Now for the way in which I have acted, it has been high-handed, and deliberately so. I have talked to three people: Turpin, the Hospital Secretary and Scott. ... Henderson for instance knows what is happening about the nerve equipment, since this is an M of H affair (he is responsible for M of H equipment).

He had not "petitioned this or that committee" – there was not time or need – and work had to go on.

> It has taken me a year to assemble the double lead electromyograph and we should not have done it without the powerful aid of the Department of Anatomy. ...
>
> This is not a confidential letter and as it is, I suppose, the only sort of answer I can give to the mischievous reports that you say are so widely circulated (how clever some people are at that sort of thing) I should be

---

89 He was writing and editing a substantial part of the report for the MRC: Zachary and Roaf 1954.

pleased if you would make its contents fairly generally known.

    My best wishes to you
        yours sincerely,
        Herbert Seddon

The Board of the Faculty of Medicine mulled over past events and considered the future:

> Those most intimately concerned with the WM hosp favour continuing the chair. ... While lamenting the failure of the Professorial Department to achieve a lasting and happy relationship with the rest of the hospital, they hold that in the academic field it was a considerable success. ... Opportunities for work have always been enough to satisfy the reasonable requirements of a professor ... but more beds, more rooms, more labs would be good. ... The late professor, as might be expected, holds other opinions. He does not believe that a Professorial unit will flourish under the conditions in which he worked 1947-48 after his Clinical Directorship was abolished, nor that minor improvements will give the Professor adequate status and powers. A similar view has been expressed by a leading orthopaedic surgeon from outside Oxford. 18 Oct 1948.

Trueta, supported by Girdlestone, was given the Nuffield chair. Seddon had advised him that, as a foreigner, he would have difficulty in achieving success. This was a red rag to a Spanish bull, and Trueta kept Seddon's letter as a challenge that he was determined to prove wrong. However, there was some truth in Seddon's advice because there was a strong old boy network among the orthopaedic surgeons, many of whom had been educated in the public school system.

When the book *Studies of Renal Circulation*, by Trueta, Barclay, Franklin and Daniel, was published that year by Blackwell, Seddon gave it a good review.[90] Fair-minded as ever, he wrote that the "book was charmingly written and superbly illustrated" and typically added a few thoughts of his own: "enlightened clinical observation may suggest experiments that not only provide the explanation of the clinical phenomenon but will, if followed with sufficient tenacity and imagination, lead into other and perhaps more important fields of inquiry."

---

90 Seddon 1948b.

Chapter 9

Return to the RNOH

Seddon welcomed the return to the Royal National Orthopaedic Hospital and the Institute of Orthopaedics as a fresh start. It was also the opportunity to realise his dream of creating a world-class centre for orthopaedics, staffed with old friends and a new generation of scientifically aware staff. Seddon's Oxford unit for peripheral nerve injuries was moved to the RNOH.

He and his family moved back into their pre-war home, Moor House, belonging to the hospital and only a short walk from there through the woods. The house was of brick, built originally in Tudor times, with additions in an Italianate style. It was very large: the drawing room housed two grand pianos and a table-tennis table easily. The garden was extensive, with lawns, shrubs and a rose garden, and it became Seddon's delight to tend it and show it off to visitors. In one corner there was an old well, surmounted by a wrought-iron arch. At last Mary did not have to share the house with her mother-in-law because Jim had found a flat for his mother in Beaumont Street in the centre of Oxford. Here she enjoyed an independent life.

Seddon had a sister, Dorothy. She was pretty and had quite a small figure. She took up nursing, rather against the wishes of her parents, and made a success of it. She had nursed at the Radcliffe Infirmary in Oxford, and in Norwich, and then became matron at the Luton and Dunstable Hospital. This was little more than 20 miles from Stanmore. Trainees from the RNOH often had to work there for a few months as part of their training. Seddon had a brother too, Ronald, the handsome favourite of his mother, who was married and, sadly, died young in a sleepwalking accident after being wounded while serving as an officer in Italy.

Seddon was an active and able administrator. He had an office in the Stanmore hospital and another at Great Portland Street. He commanded respect from his surgeons, but also fear – he could be quite sharp. On the wards he was seen in a white coat, like all

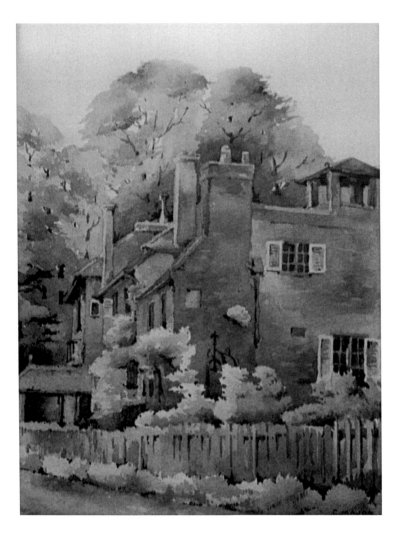

15. Water colour of Moor House by a friend of the Seddons

medical staff, and a bow tie, like many surgeons, particularly
paediatricians. Matron, sisters, nurses and ward orderlies could all be
instantly recognised by their distinctive uniforms. Two or three days
a week, Seddon descended into the smoke and traffic of central
London to work at the Institute of Orthopaedics in Great Portland

Street as Director of Studies. Jackson Burrows had already been appointed Dean.

The waiting area for the clinics in Bolsover Street had been decorated with frescos when Seddon was resident surgeon at Stanmore. They portray the months of the year, each with a beautiful maiden involved in some seasonal activity, and were created by Nan West, a student from the Slade School of Art.[91] An additional painting of a tea party, complete with uniformed waitress, in front of the white cliffs (of Dover?) was symbolic of the British way of life and middle-class values. They impressed patients with an atmosphere of calm grandeur as they awaited an appointment with the consultant and his junior staff.

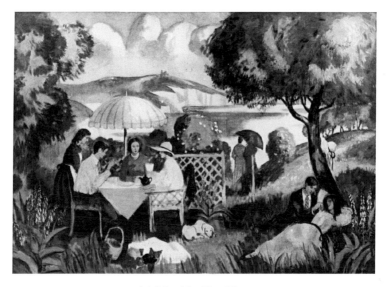

16. Mural by Nan West

One patient remembers his mother trembling with awe in the waiting hall in Bolsover Street and sitting there for several hours until they were seen. Seddon, surrounded by younger doctors, leaned forward and in a kindly tone asked "How are you getting on?" He remembered or had made a note that the boy was a keen cricket player – "five wickets for 25 runs" – but now it was even better: six

91 Shott 1998.

wickets for 10 runs. Seddon turned to his secretary and told her to make a note of that! That patient went on to study medicine when he grew up and worked for Seddon as an SHO (senior house officer).

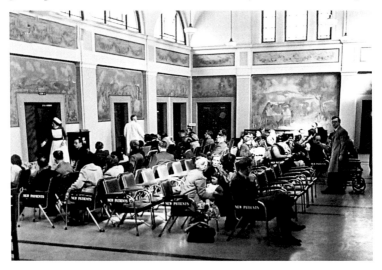

17. Bolsover St Hall 1965

Setting up and running a new department, teaching, operating and undertaking research must have left little time to write. In the evening he might be heard speaking into a dictaphone while in the background the family cocker spaniel barked and Sally might be heard practising piano. Seddon's personal pet was a Siamese cat.

Among the archives of University College is some history of the origin of the RNOH and the Institute:

> Although many of the leaders of British Orthopaedics had received their training at the Royal National Orthopaedic Hospital (RNOH), there was no formal school set up before 1946. The RNOH was recognised as a postgraduate teaching hospital and it was recommended that an Institute of Orthopaedics should be founded and that it should be associated with the RNOH.

The Institute of Orthopaedics & Musculoskeletal Science (IOMS) was founded at the RNOH in the Summer of 1946, initially located at the RNOH site in Great Portland Street, London. Stanmore in Middlesex, the country branch of the hospital, offered better facilities for expansion and by 1948 most of the Institute facilities had moved to Stanmore.

Retiring from the Nuffield Professorship of Orthopaedics in Oxford in 1948 Mr Herbert Seddon occupied the post of Director of Studies as a joint appointment between the RNOH and the Institute.

The RNOH was now a National Health Service hospital and there were other changes since Seddon had last worked there. He had been in America at the beginning of the war when the Emergency Medical Service had decided to evacuate the RNOH patients to Scotland and move the staff and patients of all London teaching hospitals to the periphery. During the war, the spacious Stanmore site became home to, among others, the Charing Cross Hospital.

Mr John Cholmeley had worked at the hospital in Stanmore since 1936, first as an assistant resident surgeon who would help with the clinics.[92] In Seddon's absence at the beginning of the war, it was he who had the responsibility, in the blackout, of getting patients in plaster and in complicated frames, their nurses and physiotherapists, plus a doctor or two all onto trains, destined first for Edinburgh and some then to other Scottish destinations. Those patients at Stanmore who were fit enough were sent home.

Then, ten days into the war, a former patient dashed upstairs to the doctors' sitting room, saying, "Mr Seddon has landed at Liverpool!" A young doctor who was there at the time tells this story and adds: "I doubt if anything in the ensuing six years caused as much immediate concern as that. We awaited his return with interest to see the outcome of the confrontation between Seddon and the Senior Surgeon of Charing Cross Hospital as to who would be boss. The answer was Seddon."[93] Even in those early days of his career, shortly before he became a professor in Oxford, he showed the ability to exert authority.

92 Kemp 1993.
93 Hulbert 1990–91.

During the war, temporary wards were erected in the grounds at Stanmore and these remained for many years. On his return there from Oxford in 1948, Seddon was reunited with some old acquaintances among the staff. The year before, as the Middlesex Hospital's consultant, Cholmeley had been occupied overseeing polio cases in the British epidemic of 1947–8; now he was working part-time, with six sessions and 60 beds at Stanmore. He remained unmarried, lived in a hospital flat and spent his spare time on cars. He was a family friend, but Sally and James had difficulty with his name and he became Uncle Tummy to them; the nickname, I am told, was apt.

Another friend was JIP James (known as Jip), who returned from a year in America, where he had studied the work being done on scoliosis in specialist centres. It was natural therefore that, when he returned, scoliosis cases should be referred to him and a unit was started at Great Portland Street. He also saw the spondolisthesis cases. Seddon thus established a trend for orthopaedic surgeons to specialise.

Philip Newman (usually called Pip) had joined the staff of the RNOH in 1946 after distinguished service in the war. He had remained at Dunkirk to care for the wounded, while others were evacuated. He started a backache clinic. A hand clinic was initiated and run by JIP James, who had also done notable service in the war among partisan guerrillas in Yugoslavia. In 1949 a leg equalisation clinic was established, with Karl Nissen in charge. Other specialist clinics added in the 1950s were for congenital dislocation of the hip, David Trevor; slipped femoral capital epiphysis, Harold Jackson Burrows; shoulder, V.H. Ellis (until his sudden death in 1953); and foot, AT Fripp. These were just a few of the surgical staff. Although they had their specialist areas they also took general orthopaedic cases. Seddon established regular lectures and clinical conferences, so forging links between the different areas of work. Occasionally his hammer fell hard, producing bright sparks and causing his junior staff to fly off to other hospitals.

Seddon saw specialisation not only as a way for surgeons to become experts in a field but also as a way of giving them time for the research he so valued.[94] He viewed private practice as a bar to

94 Seddon 1961a.

doing useful research; he personally had almost no private patients. Newman, Trevor and Nissen came to the RNOH at the same time as Jackson Burrows, who was the first Dean of the Institute of Orthopaedics and played a key part in its development.

The precious records of peripheral nerve injuries were defended by an Olympic fencer, Mrs Mary Glen Haig. There were some people in Oxford who argued that they should not have been removed. They were preserved until the 1990s, when an order from the Dean of the Institute for their destruction was countermanded by Professor George Bonney. He and the RNOH photographer, Mr Cook, who had been alerted to the loss of the archive, saved the best of them and transferred them to St Mary's Hospital.

When Seddon's peripheral nerve injury unit moved to the RNOH in London, Donal Brooks came too. Donal has been described as a "deft and precise operator who treated tissue with respect and reaped the reward of this care".[95] In addition to being a good surgeon, he was witty and had "a warm agreeable manner, charm and imperturbability". Maybe it was that imperturbability that caused him and Seddon to be likened to Jeeves and Wooster. Seddon was full of admiration: "the elegance of his operative technique is of an order I have never been able to achieve". Donal (or Don) certainly had style; he had an estate in County Limerick and drove an old Bentley, whereas the Seddons had a practical, if upmarket family car, a good solid Rover 90. Don Brooks was to see and investigate all cases of poliomyelitis; in May 1948 he was made a consultant at Stanmore with particular responsibility for physiotherapy and rehabilitation. Later he became one of "the best and greatest pioneers of British hand surgery" with consulting rooms in Harley Street.

John Daniel had been a part-time rehabilitation officer and he was now made full-time. In addition to providing physical rehabilitation, the hospital would have had a lady almoner – as a social worker was then called – but there was no specialist in mental rehabilitation and no psychiatry at the hospital. Advice was of the type given by Seddon to the Dutch airman: "He warned me strongly not to take painkillers, alcohol and any other sedative. He advised me to keep myself bodily as well mentally fit. To keep one goal in life based on the future, making good use of knowledge and experience gained

---

95 Bonney 2004.

during life."

The plaster technician was another important member of the team that treated the patient. Plaster of Paris was heavy and had to be applied wet. Seddon and the staff co-operated in some research at the Institute using "polythene". Polyethylene had been synthesized in 1933 by ICI and had been used by the military in the war. It was now manufactured by Du Pont under the name Polythene and became widely available. A study of 'The use of polythene and resinated asbestos felt for splints' was published in 1950.[96]

In addition to peripheral nerve injuries, Seddon became a recognised expert on the brachial plexus.[97] In the triangle between neck and shoulder there is a complex tangle of important nerves, arteries, veins and other structures. Five nerve roots from the spine combine to form the brachial plexus. From there, three nerves go down into the arm: the median, the ulnar and the radial. For the purpose of recovery, it was important to know whether the injury was pre- or post-ganglionic. Seddon observed several features that were only occasionally found: firstly, myelinated axons in the peripheral nerves of the affected limb; secondly, the operative finding of apparently undamaged plexus; and thirdly, the demonstration of ganglion cells in the plexus. This prompted research by Bonney and others.

However, in later years, as Rolfe Birch points out, "the RNOH did not take on the challenge of the injury to the brachial plexus, nor it did not absorb the one important lesson from 'microsurgery', which is that small arteries can be successfully repaired so that amputated hands can be reattached or flaps of vascularised skin or bone or even nerve can be used in the reconstruction of damaged limbs.'

Bonney and his colleagues proposed[98] that the damage to the proximal limb of the axon of the dorsal root ganglion would not affect the distal axon or its myelin sheath. The first experiments[99] studied the axon reflexes evoked by an intradermal injection of histamine and by exposure of the digits to cold water, in a series of patients with injuries to the peripheral nerves or to the brachial

---

96 Scales 1950.
97 Seddon 1948c, 1949.
98 Birch, Bonney & Wynn 1998, Chapter 9.
99 Bonney 1954.

plexus, or after cervico dorsal sympathectomy.

The injury was assessed with a 'triple response' test of histamine reaction to stimuli, which included dipping fingers in warm water. Mylograms also could give information. Seddon formulated the method of treatment, but the operations were not very successful. Philip Yeoman wrote a thesis on injuries to the brachial plexus, and he and Seddon published 'Brachial plexus injuries: treatment of the flail arm' in 1949.[100] Some of the injuries were caused by badly adjusted backpacks, some as a result of falls from motor cycles and others by various diseases.

Seddon also treated cases of Pott's disease. Pott's paraplegia is a condition induced as a result of spinal tuberculosis: pressure on the spinal cord from an abscess results in paralysis, as Seddon had shown many years before. Drain the abscess, halt the infection and the patient had a good chance of recovery. Gaining access to the infected area was a long and difficult procedure, and several surgeons worked to perfect an operation using an antero-lateral approach.

Under Seddon's auspices, the organic and scientific aspects of medicine were developed. A metabolic unit (Ward 2 at Stanmore) was started under Reginald Nassim and in April 1949 a morbid anatomist and a biochemist were appointed to the pathology department for both the institute and the hospital. The need for radiographs to be accurately reported had been pointed out to the Medical Staff Committee by Campbell Golding, a radiologist who had sessions at the RNOH and the Middlesex. As a result, three part-time radiologists were appointed. Seddon asked one of them, RO Murray, to give regular tutorials to the orthopaedic registrars. Murray and the orthopaedic surgeon AT Fripp built up a collection of photographs and radiographs that later, with Campbell Golding's collection, became the nucleus of the film museum at the Institute of Orthopaedics.[101]

One of the Stanmore hospital physicians, Harwood Stevenson, and his wife Frances became close friends with the Seddons. There is a story about him, told by Ross Nicholson:

---

100 Yeoman and Seddon 1961.
101 Stoker 1995.

It happened that Harwood Stevenson was asked for an opinion. A lengthy and detailed report over his name came back, to be followed later the same day by an identical report over the name of the registrar. HJS read this and he dictated the note: 'See Matthew, Chapter 6 Verse 7 – vain repetition'. This of course reads 'use not vain repetition, as the heathen do: for they think that they shall be heard for their much speaking'.

Colonel EK Wood had been appointed before the war as Superintendent of the newly built training college. Subsequently he was made secretary of the hospital. He had served in the Indian Army and was recalled in the second war, serving in Iraq and India. Like the Seddons, he lived in a hospital house – Limes Farm House was near the training college at the western end of the hospital grounds. After the war he was appointed House Governor and and Secretary.

Although the hospital was now funded by the government, additional support was raised by charitable efforts. In those days the hospital had some community life, such as a Christmas pantomime. It was expected that a head of department would entertain his staff during the year; Seddon, being paternalistic and concerned with the welfare of the young surgeons, enjoyed these occasions. He and Mary entertained all the registrars to lunch or dinner at Moor House. John and Gwyneth Chalmers, who were at RNOH in the 1950s, remember a very happy and relaxed Christmas party. They were surprised when their austere director transformed the dining table with a blow football set and threw himself into the game like a small boy. He so rarely allowed this sense of fun to show. In the summer the Chalmers family escaped to a very isolated cottage at Clashnessie on the west coast of Scotland for their holiday, they were amazed one day to see Seddon striding across the hill. He just thought he would drop in and see how they were.

Many surgeons devise their own instruments and Seddon used a needle holder of his own design. There is a photograph of the simple instruments he used in peripheral nerve surgery:

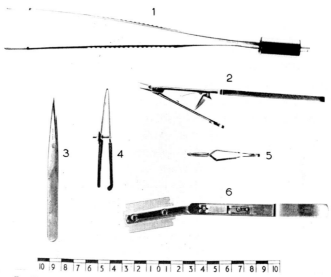

FIG. 15, 19. Instruments used in nerve suture.

18. Simple instruments Seddon used in peripheral nerve surgery
Fig 15 from *Surgical Disorders of the Peripheral Nerves*

1.Bipolar stimulator: a smaller model is often
convenient
2.Ophthalmic needle holder
3.Watchmaker's forceps
4.Crile's arterial clamp for controlling the circulation
in a nerve
5.Carrel's arterial clamp, used for securing the first
two stitches in suture of a nerve
6.Razor-blade holder.

In the operating theatre, Seddon was meticulous about
preparation by his staff; for example, when towelling up, the towels
had to be folded back exactly so many inches. Treating patients was
a serious business and there was no place for idle chat. His mood was
one of concentration; if vexed, he might say 'damn' but he would not
really swear. When he handed over to his assistant and left the the-

atre, the atmosphere lightened and there would be some banter, particularly with the nurses. He was a good operator. His operating technique was interesting because he was completely ambidextrous and it was a challenge to the registrar assisting to know from which direction the next action would come. When the registrar was permitted to do a procedure, if it was taking too long or was not quite right, Seddon would impatiently tap with whatever instrument he was holding, and this was a sure sign of imminent sharp criticism.

Peripheral nerve operations were very time-consuming. When he had a trained assistant, Seddon would spend two hours in theatre and then, having exposed the nerve, would leave the assistant to join the nerve, complete the operation and sew up. The whole operation might take as much as five hours.

In 1946 the role of the institute was described as first to train orthopaedic surgeons for the NHS and second to teach orthopaedic surgery, also running refresher courses for general practitioners alongside courses for school medical officers and FRCS exam candidates. The obituaries of Herbert Seddon published in 1978 give some good descriptions of life in the new department.

More personal memories come from Ross Nicholson, who says of Seddon that

> From the time he came back to RNOH in 1948 and through the 1950s in particular, RNOH was the preferred centre in the UK for New Zealand graduates. There were usually five or more in house officer or registrar posts. In those days, the career path was to obtain the English Fellowship, in General Surgery, it being the only option, and then to train further in orthopaedics before returning home.

Ross spent six months at Great Portland Street in 1951, but it was when he returned four years later that he really saw the way Seddon worked.

> After a couple of years, I felt the desire to return to RNOH. On inquiring about possible jobs, I received what I later realised was the usual response, that there

were no registrar posts available, and perhaps I would like to work as a house officer. I accepted and started at Stanmore in 1955 on the Seddon Team but also working with other consultants.

I was well aware that, on the first ward round, the new house surgeon was destined as it were to be put in his place. I had worked very hard to work up the patients. On being asked of one patient who had not been discharged, I told HJS that this was "because of her home circumstances". The response "What circumstances?" illustrated his ability to ask the next question, and not just accept what one has been told. This episode alone has influenced me all my practising life.

I was required to make up the operation list after that first ward round and did so with great care. Next morning HJS's first greeting was: "You have altered the operation list". I remonstrated that I was sure that I had not, and he was equally adamant. He agreed we would wait until the next ward round, when he could check on the notes that he had dictated. In due course he checked the notes, looked at me across the patient's bed, a slight incline of the head and simply "You were correct". There was no apology, and indeed even now, I did not expect one, but it was apparent that I had made my mark.

HJS was technically excellent at every procedure he undertook. This included arthrography of the hip in those with congenital dislocation. Remember that there were no image intensifiers in those days, and there were tricks for knowing when one was in the joint, even before the x-rays were taken. HJS had become significantly deaf by that time, but did have one ear more affected. This allowed for 'asides' between members of the team, but I suspect that sometimes the old man in fact heard these. On this particular day, there was great difficulty with the arthrogram. The x-ray was taken and John Hall said to me: "It looks as though some of the dye has leaked into the hip joint". There was no comment from HJS, and although it would be going too far to say that he threw the syringe on the table, he certainly planted it firmly and walked out.

One Saturday a patient was admitted acutely with an incomplete paraplegia, from tuberculosis of the spine. John and I took a very careful history, did a detailed examination, testing and muscle charting most carefully. We then called in HJS who, as was his wont, checked our findings, calling out his gradings and comparing them with ours. To our absolute consternation we were poles apart, and I was feeling incompetent and useless. However, HJS turned to us and said "I have seen this before, with improvement occurring after the patient has been lying flat for a time." Sighs of relief but another demonstration of his clinical acumen and experience.

One day we were invited to Moor House for a sherry after work. These invitations had a reputation among the staff as the occasions for telling those invited, either that they needed more time in general surgery, or that orthopaedics was not for them. This was more than ever likely if you were asked to view the rose garden. We had a most pleasant time and were about to leave, when HJS said: "Would you like to see the rose garden?" This passed off uneventfully, apart from the fact that we both had almost uncontrollable fits of giggling, which must have made HJS wonder what was going on.

It was only after a few weeks that John Sharrard who had the post later to become known as "first assistant" left to take up his consultant post in Sheffield. One weekend there was a cricket match between the medical staff and the consultants. I was not playing, and HJS was fielding on the boundary. Between overs, he came up to me and said: "Would you like to take John Sharrard's job?" I accepted with alacrity. It is interesting to look back on the lack of formality in those days, and the way in which one could be chosen for a plum job.

At that time Lorden Trickey [later Dean of the Institute] was the RSO at Stanmore. He was by far the most knowledgeable of the registrars at that time, and we spent many hours viewing x-rays and discussing cases in the evenings. HJS had carried out a biopsy of a patient with an L4 vertebral lesion. The histology showed nothing abnormal, and a check x-ray showed that the wrong level had been operated on. Lorden and I discussed at length how we would break the news to HJS. We had already told the patient, and worked out that if I started telling him halfway between the children's wards and the huts, that I would break the news just as we arrived at the ward. The conversation went something like this.

"Sir, remember that patient with the L4 lesion?"

"Of course I do."

"The histology report shows no abnormality."

"Oh."

"X-ray shows that the biopsy was of L3."

"My dear chap, you don't mean to tell me?"

We entered the ward – I still recall that the patient was in the second bed on the left. HJS simply said:

"My dear, we biopsied the wrong level. We will have to do it again. At least we will know our way in." The patient accepted this calmly. HJS's honesty and acceptance of the mistake, without attempting to blame anyone else, indicates another outstanding facet of his character.

In the operating theatre, one assisted him with nerve repairs. After a few cases, he would assist you, and then would leave you to carry out the actual suture of the nerve. His operation notes were meticulous in their detail, but never superfluous. The note would conclude: "and then DRN did a very nice suture". However, enquiry would show that he did not assume this, but had asked the theatre sister.

As one's competence and experience increased, he would say: "I would like you to do the list this afternoon – I will be in the building". It was certainly comforting to know that he was available. The day then came when he asked me to do the list. When I asked, "You will be in the building?" the reply was "I will not." This supervised and graduated approach to training also greatly influenced my practice and registrar training. HJS's ability, not only to show confidence in young people, but also to give them confidence was another trait.

His confidence also extended beyond the operating theatre. I wanted to go to Oxford to view a research project on muscular redevelopment after polio. HJS was going on MRC business, and we decided to go together. I reported to Moor House in my pre-war Ford 8 and we drove off in his Rover 90 with me driving. At that time it was my ambition to have such a car one day, and if I did, I felt that I would have arrived. It was an anxious time driving to Oxford, but I was then told that he would be staying overnight to visit his mother, and I would drive the car back to London, while he returned by train. No need to say that the drive back alone was more of an ordeal than having HJS in the passenger seat, but it did show confidence in me.

He had a very quick mind and could be incisive in his comments. If I recall, on a Grand Round he asked George Bonney if he could do a sweat test on a brachial plexus injury and George replied: "It would be possible today sir, and practicable tomorrow." The response was: "Yes, George, but when would be preferable?"

George Bonney was bonny by nature as well as by name. He had qualified at St Mary's and trained in orthopaedics at the RNOH. Rolfe Birch tells this story about him:

Seddon summoned George Bonney and invited him to go out and found an orthopaedic department. George Bonney was very pleased about this and asked where the department might be:

"Calcutta."
"Can you not make it further, Sir?"

For most of Seddon's life, Britain had a huge empire and to him it was nothing unusual for a young man to be posted to its far reaches; but now independent India would send its own graduates for further training in Britain. So it was that Bonney left the RNOH to found the orthopaedic and fracture service at Southend Hospital where he worked single handed before coming back to join John Crawford Adams at St Mary's in 1955. In the future, that orthopaedic department became *the* centre of excellence, recognised nationwide for treatment of injuries to the brachial plexus.

To return to Ross Nicholson's memories. One day Jip James opined on a grand round that a certain condition was common and, having been challenged, was saved by HJS saying:

> "Perhaps, Mr James, we could say that it is common in the British Museum."
>
> At times when dealing with registrars who did not meet his expectations, he could be cutting, but I must say his comments were never undeserved. I recall one registrar being told: "Do you mean to say that you have worked here for two years and learned nothing?"
>
> During my time with HJS, Donal Brooks was away for several months doing trauma in Glasgow, in order to fulfil the job specifications for a consultant post designed for him – as Don commented, the only thing it didn't say was "must be Irish and have blue eyes". This meant that not only did I have considerably more responsibility, but I also had considerably more hands-on experience.
>
> To many of the junior staff HJS, I know, seemed remote. However, the closer one worked with him, the more one came to respect him.

Ross Nicholson published a paper[102] jointly with his boss in 1957, shortly after leaving Stanmore.

> On leaving RNOH I asked him if he would autograph my copy of the MRC Report on Peripheral Nerve Injuries of which he was the editor. As I passed it to

102 Nicholson and Seddon 1957.

him, he asked: "Where did you get this?" I suspect he thought I was souveniring one of the Department's copies, but when I told him that I had bought it at the Stationery Office, he wrote in his elegant hand "To O.R.N., a souvenir of a happy and profitable association. H.J. Seddon, November 1956".

Unfortunately he never visited New Zealand, but his influence, and that of the other consultants at RNOH, on New Zealand orthopaedics can never be overestimated.

Chapter 10

National celebrations, international expert

In 1947 the government began making plans to celebrate the centenary of the Great Exhibition of 1851. Something was very much needed to lift the spirits of the British people, for whom peace had not brought prosperity but rationing and austerity. A bitterly cold winter combined with fuel shortages, mostly coal but also paraffin, made conditions harder. The whole population had been enrolled into the war effort. Now, what jobs there were had to be redistributed as the demobilised forces returned to civilian life.

London was still pockmarked with bomb craters and demolished buildings because reconstruction was frustrated by shortages of building materials and many delays. One site of extensive damage was on the south bank of the Thames next to Waterloo Bridge. Plans were made to transform this area into the site of the Festival of Britain, a celebration of the British Isles, its people and achievements from ancient times to the present. A new concert hall with superb acoustics was also to be built, and Seddon's children were excited at the prospect. Sally and James were both musical and Sally was later to make a career as a professional pianist.

Teams of designers worked on the whole event. Every detail of the Festival of Britain was carefully discussed. The Typographical Panel was chaired by Charles Hasler, who had been appointed an exhibition designer for the Ministry of Information and the Central Office of Information in 1942 and had worked on displays such as Dig For Victory, Make Do and Mend, and The Nation and the Child.

In 1951 the complex of exhibitions was opened and people flocked to see what was inside. British medicine had plenty to show. Among other things, the Dome of Discovery illustrated the rapid changes in medicine and surgery that had come in the post-war period. One area was devoted to advances in tropical medicine; another showed the role modern drugs had played in the reduction of malaria and sleeping sickness, and it was hoped in curing leprosy; in another pavilion, topical subjects were selected for display. There were charts showing the reduction in death rates as a result of diphtheria immunisation and descriptions of how biological standards for drugs were being established. The importance of penicillin in saving life was given due prominence.

People could wonder at the machinery first used to produce penicillin in quantity, an extraordinary contraption using milk churns. Other machines on show were Professor Adrian's EEG (electroencephalograph) for detecting and charting electrical brain waves and an ECG (electrocardiograph) machine. This was complemented by the work of Lewis and Mackenzie on heart beats and the pulse. Of surgery, some classical instruments revised by great British surgeons were shown and also modern instruments. British anaesthesia was said to lead the world. There was also a model showing the first blood transfusion.

Six British industries were featured in the Power and Production Hall: woodworking; rubber and plastics; glass; textiles; pottery; and papermaking and printing. Visitors were able to see that precious commodity paper actually being made, out of a kind of porridge that was spread on to wire racks.

In the spring of 1950, in preparation for the Festival, the Secretary of the Royal Society of Medicine wrote to the Orthopaedic Section Secretary to suggest "A symposium designed to attract medical men from overseas attending the Festival should be arranged for May [1951], and a special summer meeting at the RNOH later in the summer" – proposals that were put into practice – and it was decided to hold a further summer meeting on 10 June at the Princess Elizabeth Hospital, Exeter. Then at the Festival of Britain meeting it was noted that Sir Harry Platt, Sir Thomas Fairbank, Sir Gordon Gordon-Taylor, Mr Bankart and Mr Watson-Jones would probably take part.

By the time the British Medical Association thought of organising a meeting, the RSM had advanced plans – details were advertised in the *British Medical Journal* on 5 May[103] – and the BMA agreed to share sponsorship. The first of the symposia, opened on

---

103 BMJ (1951) **1** 1033.

Monday 4 June by the Chancellor of the University of London, Major General the Earl of Athlone, and chaired by Sir Henry Dale, was sold out. Seddon (one of seven speakers including JZ Young and Graham Weddell) presented "Recent advances on the repair of injured nerves" and the following Monday he spoke on "Poliomyelitis: the convalescent stage" in which he protested that treatment should be realistic and simplified, and that it was important to exercise the muscles. This meeting was followed by one in Stanmore chaired by AT Fripp. Here Seddon's topic was "Antero-lateral decompression of Pott's paraplegia".

Surgeons on the organising committee of the English-Speaking Orthopaedic Associations were inspired to have their third joint meeting in London with post-conference tours to various centres including Edinburgh. As well as the academic content, luxurious entertainment was planned for the delegates.[104] E & S Livingstone no doubt had a presence at the London conference and then in Edinburgh to advertise their medical textbooks.

The process of reviewing the surgery and treatment of war casualties continued for several years in the UK and USA. In 1949 the *British Journal of Surgery* published a supplement on war surgery. Herbert Seddon and George Riddoch contributed a chapter on 'Surgery of peripheral nerves'.[105] War injuries were often extensive and the control of infection by the newly developed agents penicillin and sulphonamides had been of great importance. The early sulphonamides had some adverse effects, and Seddon warned of the severe consequences following the accidental injection of sulphonamides into the sciatic nerve.

The Medical Research Council in 1954 published a report on treatment of nerve injuries. Seddon was an editor and contributor.[106,107] The report began with details of the headings for case notes that George Riddoch had wanted to become the standard for all centres. The Oxford Centre had added headings for operation notes (Section I Part I, Methods of investigating nerve injuries; Section IX, Nerve grafting and other unusual forms of nerve repair).

---

104 Editorial, JBJS 1952.
105 Seddon and Riddoch 1953.
106 *See* Appendix.
107 Seddon 1954.

Professor Rolfe Birch, present-day editor of the book that Seddon had been invited to write for E & S Livingstone, has pointed out that the chapter

> which relates to grafting is particularly important, for in it he sets out the indications, the techniques and the results of a number of methods including the use of strands of nerves of cutaneous sensation, which is now [in 2010] the convention, of sections of main nerves, and of the "pedicle" graft which was invented by Roland Barnes and Derek St. Claire Strange. This last method is the forerunner of the free vascularised nerve graft.

The Oxford Unit had had 68 per cent success with homo-grafts, but heterografts failed. Peter Medawar, of Nobel Prize fame, who was one of JZ Young's team, suggested that it was due to an immune reaction.[108]

In Section II Part I, Lesions in continuity, Zachary and Roaf gave the interesting statistic that "The incidence of lesions to the radial nerve came third after that of median and ulnar nerves in British casualties in World War II".[109] Seddon had a series of 379 cases of median and ulnar nerves damaged by missiles, in 70 per cent of which the nerves had been divided or partly divided.

The breadth of Seddon's expertise was often demonstrated. At the British Orthopaedic Association's Spring 1951 meeting in Cambridge, during a symposium on congenital dislocation of the hip, he gave a review of treatment carried out at the RNOH over the first forty years of the twentieth century. He also briefly mentioned some work he had done with a surgeon from Ceylon, GM Muller.[110]

Also at that meeting was a distinguished professor from Paris, Merle d'Aubigné. The d'Aubigné and Seddon families had become friends in Seddon's Oxford days. In 1955 a joint meeting with the French Association of Orthopaedics was held in Paris, and in 1956 an Anglo-French scholarship brought Ann Segal to the institute, where she studied paralysis of the elbow. In 1959 she was first author of a paper with Seddon and Brooks.[111] When Merle

---

108 Young 1993.
109 Zachary and Roaf 1954.
110 Muller and Seddong 1953: re. screening of neonates.

d'Aubigné's multi-author work *Chirurgie orthopédique des paralyses* appeared in 1957, Seddon reviewed it for the *Journal of Bone and Joint Surgery*.[112] He wrote that "One of the happiest features of the book is the balanced account it gives of French, American and British practice", adding that it was pre-eminently Merle d'Aubigné who had developed the "splendid relationship between French and English orthopaedic surgeons".

In Dublin for the BOA's 1953 Spring meeting, Seddon, Lloyd Griffiths and Roaf held a joint discussion on Pott's paraplegia and its operative treatment. This was the first public appearance of work that was published a few years later, provoking anger in Macmillan, who was still waiting for that book on peripheral nerve injuries.

In 1954 Seddon attended the Sixth Congress of the International Society of Orthopaedic Surgery and Traumatology, another opportunity to make foreign contacts. At such meetings, Seddon would often add a word or two to discussion on subjects as diverse as surgical measures for the relief of paralysis of the intrinsic muscles of the toes or treatment of innocent nerve tumours by enucleation. He also added to his list of publications.[113]

There were also meetings of the RSM Orthopaedics section. At one of these in 1948 a film was shown from Ramshoff's department in America, demonstrating a new way of treating acute poliomyelitis with injections of curare (Intercostin). Seddon missed nothing and got up to speak. He said he had visited the clinic, but had not seen curare in use. He observed that the agonised expressions shown in this film were disturbing; he doubted the efficacy of the drug and thought it was actually the determination of the physiotherapists that was getting the success, adding that exercise should begin only after the acute phase had passed. Seddon was not afraid to speak up when an emperor had no clothes.[114]

Seddon was elected President of the Orthopaedic Section of the RSM and gave his presidential address to 126 fellows, members and visitors on 1 February 1949 at 8.30 p.m. at Wimpole Street. He spoke on 'The practical value of peripheral nerve repair', illustrated by a demonstration of cases. Among them was the medical student from Worcester College, Oxford (p. 90). The subject chosen for the

---

111 Segal, Seddon and Brooks 1959.
112 Seddon 1957a.
113 Seddon 1952.
114 Seddon 1948d.

AGM and Symposium was reconstructive surgery of the paralysed upper limb. Professor Robert Merle d'Aubigné (Paris) gave a paper, Seddon gave one on 'Transplantation of pectoris major for paralysis of flexors of the elbow' and Don Brooks also spoke.[115] The June meeting was held at Roehampton, and then at Wimpole Street on 4 October Norman Capener was inducted as the new president. Seddon joined VH Ellis and George Perkins as a vice-president.

In 1953 *Poliomyelitis* by Russell was published. William Ritchie Russell was a consultant neurologist who worked with Sir Hugh Cairns from 1948. He was another of the leading figures of Oxford medicine known to Seddon, who gave his book a candid review.[116]

> Serious doubts, such as I myself must feel, about Ritchie Russell's views on the treatment of a paralysed weak muscle, should not blind us to the merits of the monograph as a whole. It is written with clarity and enthusiasm; it should help us all, in the new responsibilities that recent epidemics have imposed … and to take a more comprehensive view of the sinister and yet fascinating scourge that threatens all civilised communities.

Seddon was very aware of the danger of infection by polio. He had rejected a proposal to create a poliomyelitis research centre in the RNOH and suggested that it should be set up in a dedicated fever hospital. As a result, the Hendon Isolation Hospital was founded.

Seddon regularly attended meetings of the BOA, which were held at centres around the country. In 1957 the association celebrated in Oswestry the centenary of Robert Jones' birth. Seddon introduced three members of the MRC Committee on Vaccination in Poliomyelitis. A session was devoted to this subject, including speakers on field trials of vaccines. In 1954 a vaccine against polio, the Salk vaccine, had been trialled in America and given to a large number of the population, but another, the Cutter vaccine, had had disastrous results, infecting patients with the virus instead of protecting them.

---

115 Brooks and Seddon 1959.
116 Seddon 1953.

With justification, people in Britain became wary of immunisation. However, successful programmes were eventually implemented in schools.

Although the number of polio cases diminished, there were still patients in iron lungs at the RNOH in 1962. Surgeons training at this time were the last to have the consequences of polio as a subject of their training course. Typical problems included were different leg lengths due to arrested growth. Tendon transplantation was one of the operations that was taught.

The turmoil of wartime Oxford and later medico-political conflicts were in the past. When Hugh Cairns died in 1952, Seddon looked back with affection to his Oxford days and remarked of his mentors Cairns and George Riddoch that "they were the best of friends a man could wish for". Gathorne Girdlestone had died in 1950, and Seddon was invited to contribute an account of his career for the *Dictionary of National Biography*. This brief life recognised the contribution to the care of cripples that Girdlestone had made with Robert Jones and his partnership with Nuffield in Oxford in establishing the Wingfield-Morris and Churchill hospitals.

It is made quite clear that Girdlestone and Seddon had very differing views – "he was not, however, a scientist and was disturbed by the growth in medicine of experimental investigation" and "essentially an autocrat, he was uncompromising and, in consequence, sometimes came into conflict with those whose ideas differed from his own" – but Seddon's generous assessment of him has survived virtually unchanged in the *Oxford Dictionary of National Biography*.

There is a story told how Seddon, needing to consult Girdlestone on some matter, asked his secretary to get the Archbishop of Canterbury on the phone. She did and then found she had an embarrassed orthopaedic surgeon talking to a confused prelate. The nickname reflected the high status of Girdlestone and was also apt because he was openly religious; in theatre he prayed aloud before wielding the knife.

Nearly a decade into his work in London, Seddon would sometimes take a rather lofty tone in answer to criticism. Let me give an example: one of his female students, with a diploma in child health, had done some research on knock knees in children, a topic suggested by Seddon. The work was published in the *British Medical Journal*[117] and was criticised in a letter. A month later, Seddon leapt to her defence in reply:

> Sir – May I ask Mr DF Ellison Nash to consider two propositions: (1) that before embarking on the treatment of a benign disorder it is usually wise to know something of its natural history, and (2) that responsibility for assessing efficacy of any particular treatment rests on those who use it rather than those who do not. If Mr Nash thinks splints are useful in the treatment of knock-knee, let him prove it – bearing in mind what has been widely recognised, and has been demonstrated by Dr AJM Morley, that the deformity usually disappears spontaneously.[118]

---

117 Morley 1957.
118 Seddon 1957b.

Chapter 11

A break with E & S Livingstone, but President of the BOA

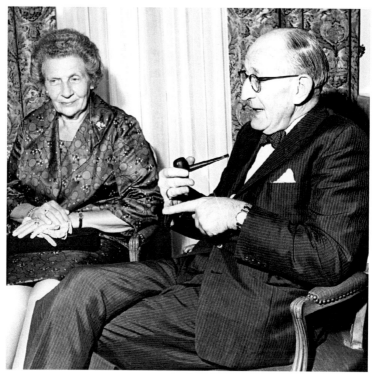

19. Jim and Mary

On 2 June 1953 people crowded round small televisions to view the coronation, broadcast live from Westminster Abbey. A friend of the Seddons, William McKie, who had been the music don at Magdalen College, Oxford, was now the organist and choirmaster at the abbey. The Seddons did not have television, but the children watched the event with Colonel Wood and his family, while Jim and Mary went into central London to join the crowds and returned soaked to the skin and fed up.

The same day the press splashed the news that the summit of Mount Everest had been successfully reached on 29 May by Hillary and Tenzing. The Seddons were particularly excited. Seddon's own climbing days were over but he still enjoyed walking. The *Times* reporter who had been with the team on the mountain was James (Jan) Morris, on his first major assignment; and the mountaineer who helped him down, inexpertly slipping and sliding, to radio the news from a Sherpa village, was Mike Westmacott. Soon afterwards Mike was introduced to Sally by a cousin and her husband Mervyn Denton, a close friend and colleague of Seddon's.

An official commemorative medal was struck for the coronation; nearly 130,000 were minted, and awarded to people in Britain and the Commonwealth. Seddon received one, and so did Mike Westmacott. His was engraved round the edge 'Mount Everest Expedition'.

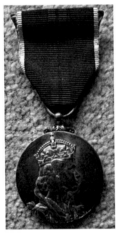

20. Coronation medal

Foreign holidays were possible and increasingly popular in the 1950s as post-war travel had become relatively easy. In 1953 the Seddons took a family holiday in France, staying at two houses that belonged to Robert Merle d'Aubigné and his Russian wife Bibka: a chalet at Argentières in the Alps, then a house in Grez-sur-Loing, an historic village south of Paris. This house had once been owned by the composer Frederick Delius and had also been home to several artists. Another year Seddon arranged for Sally, who was at school at North London Collegiate, to spend time with the family of a French orthopaedic surgeon, Hussenstein. Meanwhile, James had won a scholarship to Charterhouse.

By this time Charles Macmillan had become an important businessman and been elected a director of Edinburgh Chamber of Commerce. Amid this success he had not quite forgotten about Herbert Seddon and that book for which an agreement had been signed so long ago, but now he heard disquieting news.

CM/SMG   14th November, 1955.

Dear Professor Seddon,

As you know, I attend regularly the Editorial Meetings of the "Journal of Bone and Joint Surgery". On Tuesday 1st November I heard Mr. Lloyd Griffiths of Manchester giving his report about the special monograph which is being prepared by Mr. Roaf of Liverpool, Mr. Lloyd Griffiths of Manchester and yourself. I was crestfallen when Mr. Lloyd Griffiths explained that already a publisher had become extremely interested and was willing to publish this work for you.

After the meeting Mr. Griffiths explained to me that evidently Mr. Cumberlege of the Oxford University Press had approached you and was extremely anxious to publish this as a special monograph in his "Modern Monographs" series. Of course, I realise that it has not yet been decided whether this work will appear in the Journal or as a special monograph and that, moreover, you can choose whom you like to publish it.

My only plea in approaching you is that during the past sixteen or seventeen years I have been extremely anxious to publish anything from your gifted pen. Perhaps you will recall the previous times I have approached you, once to do an authoritative textbook with two senior editors, Sir Harry Platt and yourself, and with Mr H. Osmond-Clarke as the junior editor.

After a great deal of correspondence this idea was temporarily shelved. The second time I approached you with a view to writing a monograph on "Diseases and Treatment of Peripheral Nerve Injuries". Actually this work had taken very definite shape and a contract was drawn up for it in 1942 but various circumstances hindered the completion of such a work, including the tragic death of Mr. W.B. Highet.

More recently I imagined that we were going to get what I have been striving after for many years, an authoritative textbook on orthopaedics. Just last week I was examining the beautiful illustrations which came from the Photographic Department of the Institute of Orthopaedics displayed at the Royal College of Surgeons in London and again I was greatly impressed by their clarity and beauty. Even when I hear that Jackson Burrows is doing another book on spinal injuries for another publisher I am still hopeful that I will get our textbook under way some time in the future.

I have always longed to have your name on our list of authors and I have stated to Mr. Griffiths that, if you come to my firm, your monograph would receive my personal care and attention and I think we could guarantee that it would be out approximately six months from the date of receiving your completed manuscript and illustration material. In fact, we might even improve on this date if the illustrations were all straightforward.

As I have stated earlier, you may please yourself and choose whichever publisher you like but I hope that, when you make your final decision you will not forget the firm of E. & S. Livingstone.

With kind regards
  I remain,
    Yours sincerely,
      Charles Macmillan.

The rebuff Macmillan received was not welcome.

BRITISH POSTGRADUATE MEDICAL FEDERATION
(UNIVERSITY OF LONDON)

THE INSTITUTE OF ORTHOPAEDICS
ROYAL NATIONAL ORTHOPAEDIC HOSPITAL
234, GREAT PORTLAND STREET
EUSton 5070   LONDON, W 1

28th November, 1955.

Charles MacMillan Esq.,
E. & S. Livingstone Ltd.,
16-17, Teviot Place,
Edinburgh, 1.

My dear MacMillan,
It was most kind of you to write to me on November 14th. I am sorry that I have not been able to reply sooner but we have suffered a grievous bereavement in my family and that has upset my programme of work.

I have known Mr. Cumberlege for a long time and have certain connections with the O.U.P. that date from my time in Oxford. I must say that greatly as I admire the productions of the House of Livingstone I think even more highly of some, though not all, of the publications of the Press. A final decision about our monograph has not been made but I must tell you frankly that I incline towards the O.U.P.

Your letter troubles my conscience. That little book on nerve injuries is still on the stocks but you will appreciate how seriously I was hindered by having to edit the report on nerve injuries for the Medical Research Council. And many other things have come in to prevent me from launching out as a medical journalist.

I have always made it clear that I could not take a leading part in the production of a textbook on orthopaedics and, so far as this hospital is concerned, we are all agreed that the responsibility for it rests with

139

Mr. Jackson Burrows and with Mr. Nissen. Alas, neither of them has done anything about it yet. I am sure you would be the first to realise that the building up of this Institute has been a strenuous task and one that has called for the active co-operation of every member of its senior staff. Although there is still much to do I think that we are reaching the stage of being established and there is some prospect of our finding the leisure that is so essential for good writing.

Yours sincerely,

H. Seddon

Macmillan was going to have to wait another decade for a book from Seddon. *Pott's Paraplegia* by DLl Griffiths, HJ Seddon and R Roaf was published by Geoffrey Cumberlege of Oxford University Press in 1956. It ran to 129 pages and was illustrated with line drawings and half-tone and colour plates. Seddon used 100 cases of Pott's disease collected between 1931 and 1934, and 75 more collected by Mr BM Hay, his senior registrar at RNOH. The book recommends antero-lateral decompression as the treatment of choice. Roaf had gained experience of treating tubercular patients in India, where long-term and elaborate treatments were not an option. Jip James described the history of Seddon's work in medical terms:

It was while at Stanmore that he made his initial contribution to the pathology of paraplegia in spinal tuberculosis. He clarified the pathogenesis of paraplegia and showed clearly that it was due to the intervertebral abscess bulging backwards against the cord, and that it was not the kyphosis that caused cord damage. He also distinguished between this early, acute paraplegia due to an abscess and late onset paraplegia due to gliosis secondary to a long-standing kyphosis and ischaemia. This understanding allowed Alexander and later Capener to develop their concept of anterolateral decompression of the cord which so fundamentally altered the outlook for these tragic patients. Seddon became highly expert in operating on these cases and

with Roaf and Lloyd Griffiths in 1956 published a
monograph, *Pott's Paraplegia*.[119]

When patients awoke from the anaesthesia and discovered that they
could once more feel even a slight breeze on their legs, it must have
been a joyful moment.

Seddon expected his junior doctors to know and have read
this book on the treatment of Pott's paraplegia. It was on one of the
ward rounds at RNOH, which were led alternately by Jip James or
Seddon, that disaster struck a young houseman. These ward rounds
were terrifying to the housemen and registrars because Seddon would
reply with withering scorn to a wrong answer and, even worse,
summon the ignoramus to his study for a little discussion afterwards.
On this particular day the question was how a patient with Pott's
should be treated and the junior replied "A laminectomy, sir". This
was an operation that was strongly contraindicated and the junior was
sacked on the spot. Seddon had that power as director. This kind of
harshness, born of a desire to achieve the highest standards, made
him very unpopular with some people. He has been described by one
who was at the RNOH in those days as a kind of Jekyll-and-Hyde
character.

In the next few years drug therapy was to almost eliminate
tuberculosis. First streptomycin was discovered. A trial of drug ver-
sus surgery was stopped short because the drug showed such good
results. When streptomycin failed, owing to the bacillus developing
drug resistance, John Crofton in Edinburgh showed how the disease
could be effectively cured by triple therapy combined with screening
any contacts of the patient. Mass X-ray picked up further cases in the
population, and tuberculosis – the 'white plague' – was conquered in
Britain. It was not expected to return, so the need to learn to operate
for Pott's paraplegia died out.

Macmillan may have felt despondent about getting a book
out of Seddon but there were plenty of other authors to keep the
firm busy. In 1956 there was the Frankfurt Book Fair to attend and
an international conference of editors in Rome and Florence. Seddon
did admire some of the E & S Livingstone books. He gave a glowing
review of *Outline of Fractures, including Joint Injuries* by John Crawford
Adams:

119 James 1978.

Mr Adams's little volume on orthopaedics was very good; this companion "Outline of Fractures" is superb ... a story to be read with enjoyment, not merely a technical synopsis ... Every now and then a short book appears which is a model of its kind. This is one of them, and its popularity ought to be such as to encourage the authors and publishers to make plans for a second edition. The cost of books is becoming a burden. Here is one of some 240 pages, elegantly printed, and only costing 27s 6d. This is good value.[120]

It also contained half-tone pictures and line drawings. Seddon's prediction that it would be a great success came true: it ran through at least seven editions over twenty years.

Seddon was busy at the hospital and at home. In 1956 the RNOH received a royal visit from Queen Elizabeth the Queen Mother. Her warmth melted the formality of the occasion, for which he wore a morning coat (Fig 22). That year Jim and Mary celebrated their silver wedding with a dinner at which John Cholmeley proposed a toast to them. Formal dress was in use again in the next year when Jim and Mary had the satisfaction of seeing Sally and Michael Westmacott marry in St John's Church, Stanmore.

For Sally and Michael's wedding there was a good family gathering, although there were not so many of the small Seddon family as there were of the Westmacotts. They spent their honeymoon at the d'Aubignés' house at Grez-sur-Loing.

One day they had lunch with the war hero Pierre Malgras in Bourges. He was a surgical friend of Jim's who had moved in 1938 from Paris to Bourges. There, by night and aided by a nurse in a secret hospital, he treated wounded resistance fighters of Arnaud de Vogues' unit. He also hid English parachutists in his home. After the war he became head surgeon in the Hotel Dieu hospital and was active in the cultural life of Bourges. He mysteriously disappeared in 1995.[121]

The Seddon family had lived in a hospital house, albeit a very attractive one, for twenty years, but Seddon had made provision

---

120 Seddon 1957c.
121 *Les Nouvelles de Bourges* (30 November 1998).

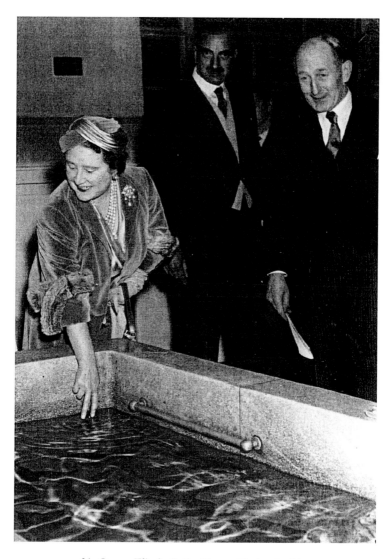

21. Queen Elizabeth the Queen Mother beside
the new therapeutic pool

for the time when he would have to, or would want to, move out by buying a nearby property called Lake House, which he rented out. Patterns of inpatient care changed and it was no longer thought necessary for senior medical staff to live at the hospital, and anyway accommodation was needed for others. Moor House was converted to house male nurses and non-medical staff. Jim and Mary moved to Lake House in 1958. It was more than big enough since their children had left home; it had a beautiful garden for Jim to care for and, as its name suggests, a small lake. By the lakeside Jim planted a rare and ancient tree from China, a meta sequoia; at the time the only other one in Britain was at Kew Gardens.

At the hospital there were new buildings, as well as changes in use of the old. Sir Henry Dale, Chairman of the Wellcome Trust, opened new research laboratories for experimental pathology in 1958. Funds for this came from the NHS and the Wellcome Foundation. Professor Charles Lack was appointed the pathologist in charge. That year Seddon was invited to give the Legg Memorial Lecture at King's College Hospital Medical School and the summer meeting of the Orthopaedic Section of the RSM was held at the RNOH. Staff there, including Seddon, demonstrated selected patients. In the afternoon Trueta was given Honorary Membership of the Section. Jip James, who had contributed so much to the rise of the Institute of Orthopaedics, left for Edinburgh where he had been appointed Professor of Orthopaedic Surgery. The return of the title of professor was something that Seddon would have to wait for.

By 1960 the decade of work that Seddon and his team had put into developing the RNOH and the institute, with the help of Jackson Burrows, was showing remarkable results. This is how Ernest Kirwan saw it:

> I first arrived as a junior in 1960 and the place was humming to the extent that it was very difficult to get any post there and everyone knew that it was a huge plus for their CV. All the British house officers had their FRCS and had to drop grades and salary in order to work there.

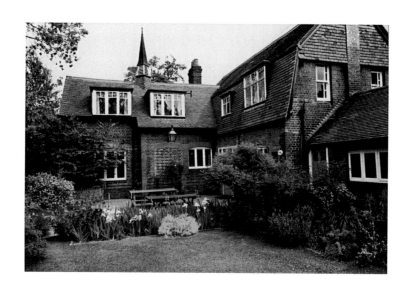

22. Lake House

They generally sat more than one FRCS – there were examinations of two Scottish colleges, the one in Dublin and the English college – thus multiplying the chances of success in these very stiff examinations. Kirwan was appointed RSO of Stanmore for three years, which meant that he worked as senior registrar and then was made a consultant at the RNOH.

Something that made RNOH "buzz" was the international atmosphere. For several years foreign physicians were given paid posts at RNOH and would stay for one or two years.. They were usually about 30 years old and came from a wide range of countries, among them Brazil, Greece, Egypt, Iraq and the Indian subcontinent. The Iraqis were often military surgeons with experience of trauma. Later, government funding for these posts was removed.

One of these international visitors was an American, DK Clawson, who was on a travelling fellowship from the National Foundation of the United States. He returned to head the Division of Orthopedics in the University of Washington. While he was in London, he and Seddon worked on the late consequences of sciatic

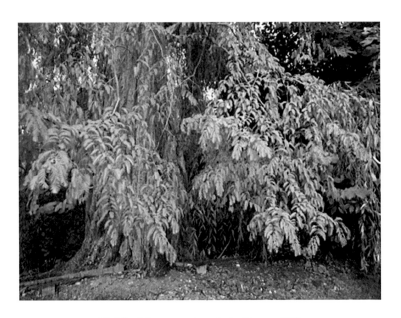

23. The Meta sequoia at Lake House 2009

nerve injury. A paper on this was presented in Chicago in 1960 and published in the *Journal of Bone and Joint Surgery*.[122] The paper begins using those three terms, neurotmesis, neurapraxia and axontmesis, thought up twenty years before and now well established. Some of the work presented had been done by Brem Highet. Closer to home, Seddon published work done with an Aberdonian, IG Mackenzie, and with David Trevor, who had made congenital dislocation of the hip his area of expertise.[123] Visitors came from the east as well as the west. The Seddon family remember with affection an Indian surgeon, Ranga Reddy, who came to Stanmore with his family.

The year 1960 was important for Seddon: he was elected president of the British Orthopaedic Association (BOA) for the year and he treated probably his most prestigious patient, Winston Churchill (see Chapter 13). The 42nd annual meeting of the BOA was held in Leeds and Harrogate. One topic discussed at that meeting was the Commonwealth Scholarship Act.

Next year, the annual meeting that marked the end of his

---

122 Clawson and Seddon 1960.
123 Mackenzie, Seddon and Trevor 1960.

presidency was a joint one with the Italian Society of Orthopaedic Surgery and Traumatology. For this, demonstrations were arranged at Stanmore. Seddon personally showed patients with Volkmann's ischaemic contraction, some cases needing muscle sliding and some tendon transplantation. Volkmann was a German physiologist; his son was a surgeon. Their observations, remembered by eponyms, were of interest to Seddon. He had published a paper about Volkmann's contracture, a condition that gives rise to a claw hand.[124] He also showed patients with Pott's paraplegia treated by antero-lateral decompression.

The American University of Beirut hosted a meeting of the Middle East Medical Assembly (MEMA) in 1961 and Seddon was among the speakers. His topics were "Nerve injuries" and "Paraplegia in tuberculous disease of the spine".[125] He had previously spent time working in Lebanon at the invitation of the army; perhaps General Iskander Ghanem, who became Commander of the Lebanese Army in 1971, was the person who invited him.

Seddon wrote an editorial for the *Journal of Bone and Joint Surgery* on an unrelated subject, congenital dislocation of the hip.[126] The issue included several papers on the subject. Seddon commented: "The conclusion is clear. A simple clinical method, easily learned and quickly applied, adding less than a minute to the time of the examination to which every new-born is entitled could take the sting out of congenital dislocation of the hip as a crippling disorder." At the Royal Society of Medicine in October, Philip Yeoman presented a paper for Seddon, a case of Leri's pleonostreosis, and again in November 1961 on *Protrusia acetabuli*.

In Edinburgh Charles Macmillan had his successes too. For twenty years the *Journal of Bone and Joint Surgery* had published papers and reported news of orthopaedic interest. It now had well over 12,000 subscribers, 7,000 of them in the United States. Charles Macmillan became chairman of the editorial board (Harry Platt had been the first, though only briefly in 1948) and arranged a celebration dinner at the Royal College of Surgeons Edinburgh on Saturday 19 December 1959. As usual, Charles kept the menu. Watson-Jones was the first editor of the journal and the finances were managed by another orthopaedic surgeon, Philip Wiles, who had a sound

124 Seddon 1956.
125 MEMA Report, III-I-5 (May 1961).
126 Seddon 1962a.

knowledge of business. Seddon remembered him for other reasons, "as a delightful companion – falling up rock faces in the Lake District and North Wales".

In 1962 E & S Livingstone's turnover was nearly twenty times that of 1944–5 and foreign sales were more than half the total, so when a new warehouse and dispatch centre was opened the next year it was very much needed. In 1963 the company celebrated their centenary with a dinner at the North British Hotel. They invited some of their most successful authors. Honorary guests were Sir Derrick Dunlop and Professor John Bruce, CBE. Charles Macmillan replied to Sir Derrick's toast with characteristic humour:

> How sweet of Professor Dunlop to make such kindly remarks about our firm. I feel it is exceedingly wise to have some of our very famous authors with us on an occasion such as this, for two reasons:-
>
> Firstly, to let those who work in the office have at least a glimpse of those very great men in Medicine. Too often all that is allotted to certain individuals is the typing out of complicated statements, and the laborious task of keeping Stock Ledgers accurately, etc, but when we see the men behind the names it makes our work far more interesting. Let me assure you, and I speak particularly to members of our staff, that even although our authors have reached such dizzying heights in the academic world they are all of them intensely human; quite a number have fascinating foibles.
>
> The second reason is to let our friends in the trade see some of the men we have got to face, those to whom so frequently we have to make our apologies when the printing, bookbinding, paper supplies, blocks etc. are delayed.

The toast of the guests was proposed by Lord Robbins and the reply was by Mr WB Hislop.

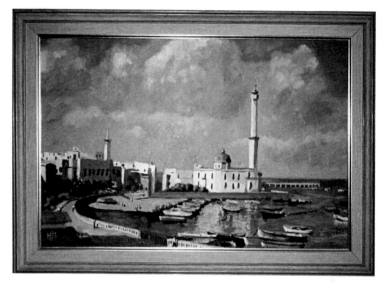

Harbour by Seddon

Chapter 12

Orthopaedics for Africa

As a young orthopaedic surgeon, Seddon had listened with admiration to Robert Jones talking about his work at a time when conditions were very different, with few medical services available to the poor. When the Manchester ship canal was being constructed, Jones had set up orthopaedic services for men who were injured. The accident rate was high and there were hardly any safety precautions. Years later Seddon compared that situation with conditions in tropical colonies, where there was still a lack of adequate orthopaedic provision. A common trauma to young men working without safety harness was injury caused by falls from coconut or clove trees.[127]

Back in 1945, Seddon had proposed that the British Orthopaedic Association should support an organisation by which orthopaedic surgeons could be seconded to the colonies for two or three years. He became a member of the Colonial Advisory Committee. In 1946, on his way back from his polio mission to Mauritius, at the request of the Kenyan Government he visited hospitals and reported on the provision of post-war rehabilitation services. He then spent a week in Uganda studying the work done in the medical school in Kampala, which had links with the University of Oxford.

He also helped to establish a panel of consultants covering a wide range of specialties in medicine, including surgery, obstetrics and gynaecology, child health, orthopaedics, tropical medicine, public health, tuberculosis, venereology and ophthalmology.[128] One of their duties was to visit Africa every three years, six of the panel going to East Africa and six to West Africa. Visiting consultants gave practical help: in 1945 Seddon had visited Nairobi; in 1948 H. Osmond-Clarke went there; in 1950 Seddon went back in September, followed by Watson-Jones in November. *The Journal of Bone and Joint Surgery* reported that "During their visits both Mr Seddon and Sir Reginald saw the work of all our departments, examined patients in the wards and out-patients, watched our surgeons operating and

---

127 Seddon 1961b.
128 *JBJS* (1951), **33** 454.

themselves did an operation, assisted by the African theatre staff."[129]

In 1942 Clifford Viney Braimbridge, a British-trained surgeon and ex-army man, started a small orthopaedic centre in Nairobi, with the help of one other young surgeon. It was successful, it grew and Braimbridge, with the Director of Medical Services, started four other centres. Seddon described the King George the Sixth Hospital in Nairobi as one of the best hospitals in the tropics and Braimbridge as the father of surgery in all Kenya. Seddon and WH Kirkaldy-Willis, who worked at the King George Sixth Hospital, described Braimbridge in an obituary as

> the perfect example of the sporting surgeon – handsome, physically in perfect trim, an ardent crick- eter, enthusiastic player of golf and tennis ... yet although he regarded surgery as a game he was determined to play it with all his might and see that others did so too. His capacity for work was prodigious – whole day operating sessions at the African hospital, week in week out ... He was a natural leader.[130]

Seddon's engagement with Africa was periodic,[131] but intense when he was there. Roy Miller, surgeon, was working in Kenya in and after the war and remembers Seddon coming out in 1950 as a travelling fellow of the Royal College of Surgeons of England. "[He] undertook a round at the Provincial Hospital at Kisumu on Lake Victoria. Characteristically, despite being orthopaedic, he saw every patient." I'm sure Braimbridge approved. "This coincided on the day x-rays became available."

Some years later, when Seddon's son James went to lecture in engineering and live in Nigeria for a while, Seddon was able to visit him. The father admired the social structure and the shared care of the extended African family, whereas his son James was more critical of how unevenly the load was spread.

---

129 *JBJS* (1951), **33** 290.
130 Seddon and Kirkaldy-Willis 1964.
131 Seddon 1959.

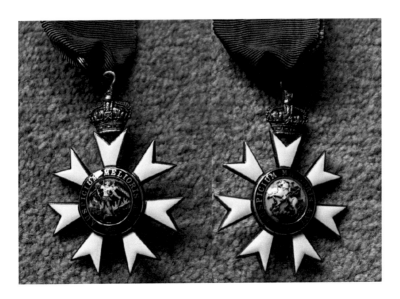

24. CMG medal, showing St Michael and St George

In the King's Birthday Honours of 1951, Seddon was appointed CMG or, to give it its full name, Commander of the Order of St Michael and St George.[132] The family went with Jim to Buckingham Palace where he received the decoration. The motto of the order – *Auspicium melioris ævi* (token of a better age) – was apt for Seddon because there were such great hopes then for the future of the colonies.

At the hospital at Mombasa, Rowland McVicker started an orthopaedic service after Kirkaldy-Willis had moved from there to Nairobi, where he concentrated on tuberculosis and polio deformities. Seddon and Robert Roaf were among the visitors.[133]

Kirkaldy-Willis collaborated with Michael Wood, a colleague at the King George the Sixth Hospital who also worked at the HH The Aga Khan Hospital in Nairobi, on a textbook of trauma surgery particularly designed for the Western-trained doctor coming to work in Africa. Their *Principles of the Treatment of Trauma, Basic Principles, Plastic and Orthopaedic Aspects of Trauma*[134] was dedicated to "The Africa Research Foundation and all who work for her". W Rainsford Mowlem and Seddon wrote forewords to the book.

132 *JBJS* (1951), **33** 454.
133 Stuart 2002.
134 Kirkaldy-Willis and Wood 1962.

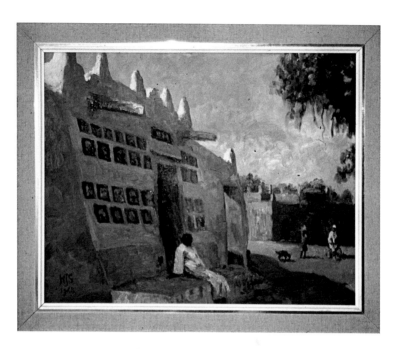

25. *Nigerian Scene* by Seddon, 1968

Mowlem began:

A first glance at the early chapters of this book could
create the impression that they are a prelude to yet
another example of high-powered surgery designed to
achieve the improbable in the face of the impossible.
Nothing could be further from the truth. The authors are
but laying the foundations of knowledge from which a
reasoned and intelligent approach can be made to everyday problems.

These are by their very nature the problems of injury,
and more particularly injury occurring to the popula-
tions in those parts of the world where surgical help is
of necessity widely scattered and where facilities are
often only basic.

Seddon described the skills needed to work as a physician in Africa:

In the hospitals of what we call advanced countries medicine has become institutionalised. An inexperienced man who has his wits about him can get along very comfortably by pulling the levers that bring this or that department into action; he may convince himself, and perhaps others, that he is competent and all this is possible with no great mental effort.

Contact with sickness and injury under primitive conditions quickly convinces a young physician or surgeon that he must bring all his powers of reasoning and all his originality to bear on the care of his patient. A modest experience of work in Africa and elsewhere taught me how little I knew of the principles, or, if the reader distrusts that overworked word, the essentials of surgical therapeutics. I have often been humbled by the astonishing range of knowledge and talent for improvisation of men and women in the district and mission hospitals of Africa and Asia. Surgeons there are general surgeons to a degree that the present generation hardly knows.

I have seen, too, the growth of excellent medical services that had their roots in the bush and in the minds of pioneers.

In 1957 Philip (Pip) Newman was sent by the Colonial Office on a seven-week tour that included Sierra Leone, the Gambia and Nigeria. He suggested sending a registrar to work with the orthopaedic specialist Arthur Frank Bryson in Nigeria. Bryson was a remarkable man, the son of a Chinese missionary, a speaker of Mandarin and a survivor of the Japanese invasion of Shanghai. Aided in part by the British Government, in 1959 Bryson founded a National Orthopaedic Hospital in Kano, northern Nigeria.

The question was how to find trained staff for the growing number of hospitals. In 1960 Seddon suggested that hospitals in the colonies might be staffed with consultants and registrars in a series of

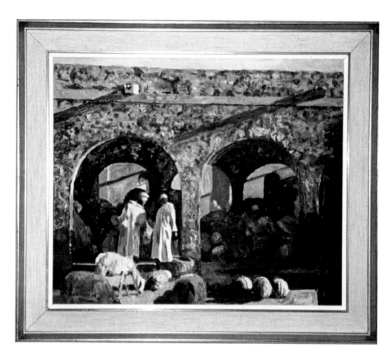

26. Kano Market by Seddon, 1969

short-term appointments on secondment from their UK posts. There was one serious drawback: at that time there were 180 registrars in the whole of the UK and this number was quite inadequate. However, there was a relative excess of senior registrars (53), who thus had to wait several years before a consultant post became available in Britain. Over ten years, 12 registrars went out to Kano for one to one and a half years each. Nursing sisters, senior and junior doctors (Derek R. Richards was the first) came in rotation from the RNOH, and Seddon was among them.[135] There they saw exotic conditions not found in London and devised simple but effective treatments wherever possible.

There was a crisis when Nigeria became independent. Bryson was offered a golden handshake and returned to Britain, leaving the visiting registrar unsupervised. The man wrote to Seddon to

135 Cholmeley 1985.

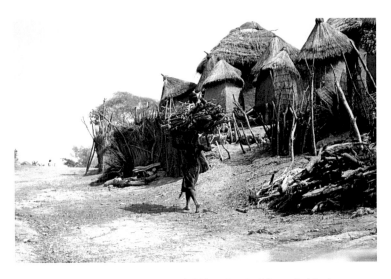

27. A scene in the town of Bida, Nigeria (photo Seddon)

ask what he should do and received the unhelpful answer "I leave it to your conscience". However, Seddon later took some action. It came about like this: Charles Manning invited him to a meeting of the Arbuthnot Lane Club, a club that Manning belonged to that organised some scientific meetings. Geoffrey Walker had worked in Kano and told members of the Arbuthnot Lane Club about the specialist orthopaedic hospital that had been built in Kano to serve a huge population; Seddon then persuaded consultants at the club to go to Nigeria for three months at a time. Thus it was that from 1963 to 1971 consultants went out to Kano from all over England, locums were found as temporary replacements and 22 consultants were seconded for three-month periods to supervise the registrars, an arrangement that was kept going all through the civil war in Nigeria.[136]

Among those who went to Kano were Bevis Brock, Brian Madden, Charles Manning, Ian Taylor, Edward Lorden Trickey, Geoffrey Walker and Ginger Wilson, along with trainees Chris Colton and Malcolm Swann. Alan Lettin and Geoffrey Walker started a club for those who had benefited from this African experience.

---

136 Waugh 1993, pp. 216–219.

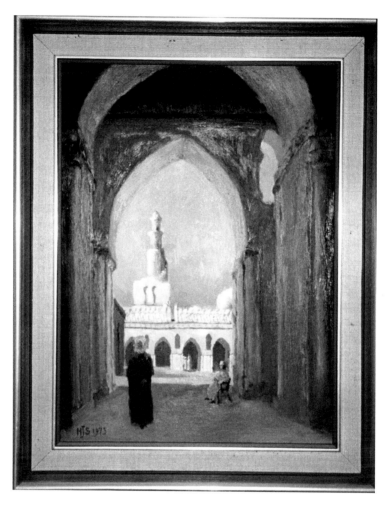

28. *Mosque* by Seddon, 1975

They named it, paradoxically, the Innominate (nameless) Club, perhaps inspired by the Lake District tarn of the same name or after the bones of the hemi-pelvis.

Seddon visited Africa in 1962 as a member of the Committee on (East African) University Needs and Priorities and again in 1964, an event reported in the *Journal of Bone and Joint Surgery*.

A symposium was held at the medical school, Makerere University College, Kampala, Uganda, from 17 to 20 March 1964, under the chairmanship of Sir Herbert Seddon, as he now was. Sponsored by the National Fund for Research into Poliomyelitis and Other Crippling Diseases, its aim was to pool knowledge and discuss problems associated with all aspects of rehabilitation in developing countries. At this time the medical school had an excellent reputation and was known particularly for tropical disease expertise.

Uganda had become an independent country in 1962 and a 1500-bed hospital, the Mulago Hospital, was built that year, but conditions in Uganda soon became more difficult. Idi Amin at that time was merely an officer in the army but he commanded the troops of the 4th KAR and was responsible for the Turkana massacre of farmers in Kenya. The British governor failed to court-martial him, and Amin gradually and violently acquired control of Uganda.

As the African countries became independent, less medical aid was provided to their medical services from Britain. However, some very important work continued in Africa and the Far East. From 1963 to 1973 Seddon chaired the MRC Working Party on Tuberculosis of the Spine and spent many hundreds of hours on its programme. A contemporary remarked that the findings of this working party were one of the outstanding achievements of the MRC and that Seddon was the driving force, mastermind and key worker of the team. Centres were selected in Korea, Hong Kong, Bulawayo and South Africa.

Seddon also served on the Colonial Advisory Medical Committee, the Tropical Medicine Research Board and the panel of colonial medical visitors.

By 1970 work in the ex-colonies had become part of third world affairs and was reported in the International Symposium on Orthopaedics in the Third World, held in Oxford.

Chapter 13

Sir Winston Churchill, statesman and patient

From the treatment of babies to that of the old, Seddon's opinion was sought. He was called in by Lord Moran to treat the great statesman Winston Churchill. Of course Seddon made handwritten case notes, which, curiously, are written in the third person in the tradition of scientific reports, but he also wrote a private account of the three accidents when he was consulted.[137]

Now this aged and corpulent statesman, who had made such a magnificent contribution to British history and led the country to victory, had suffered several strokes and was nearing the end of his life.

Here are some extracts from Seddon's typed account (now in the RCS) and letters (in the Churchill Archives, Cambridge).

1960 Fracture of the thoracic spine

Just after midnight, 15-16th November, Sir Winston slipped in Lady Churchill's room when he went to say goodnight to her, sat down heavily and banged the back of his head against a wall. He was badly shaken but they managed to get him into bed, and Lord Moran came to see him. He could not find any localizing signs because Sir Winston said he felt sore all over. There was no bruising at the back of the head or elsewhere.

He telephoned me in the morning, I went to Hyde Park Gate at 11.45 and found Sir Winston propped up in bed and very comfortable. There was a small swelling at the back of his head but nothing else. A little tenderness at the upper end of the thoracic spine but no other abnormality. I telephoned Campbell Golding [the leading orthopaedic radiologist of the time, who was on the staff of the RNOH] who told me that x-rays of the upper thoracic spine taken with a portable machine would be useless; we would have to go to his consulting room.

---

137 MSO279, RCS Eng.

Trying to wrap up Sir Winston produced such violent pain in the upper thoracic spine that we had a bit of a game getting him down the stairs and into the ambulance. I held Sir Winston's head firmly during the journey, but he still had a good deal of pain. Golding took x-rays of the thoracic spine and of the pelvis and we found a crush fracture with no displacement of T5.

I would have liked pictures of the cervical spine too, but Golding said it would be necessary for him to sit on a stool; this was out of the question because it would have hurt him so much. Anyway there was nothing to suggest a fracture in the neck.

Lord Moran and I agreed to nurse him at home with day and night nurses from St Mary's Hospital.

17.11.60 Sir Winston had been fairly comfortable sleeping on his back, but Lord Moran told me that this position would almost certainly be fatal; his chronic bronchitis made his chest like a musical box. He must be sat well up. So I ordered a hospital bed that we could crank up. Later in the day Philip Yeoman and I – purposely avoided saying to Sir Winston what we had in mind – lifted him smartly into the sitting position and moving him into the new bed. The patient expressed his views about us in the strongest possible terms, ending with a growl "Narrow beds – narrow minds". We could not have avoided hurting him, but the pain soon subsided and we never had another cross word.

18.11.60. A very busy day starting with a telephone call at 6 a.m. To the effect that Sir Winston had wakened with pain in the right shoulder radiating to the sternum. One or other of us made visits during the day and the last one was by Lord Moran, John Richardson and myself at 8.45 p.m. Richardson did an E.C.G. Tracing. Fortunately, he had one that had been done in June; he found no change at all and the physicians concluded that there had been no serious cardiac episode in the night. However, the patient was still bothered by pain in the neck and in both shoulders. I knew he had dislocated the right one when he was young and it would not abduct beyond 90°. At one point Lord Moran, John Richardson and I found ourselves standing in a row before Sir Winston, telling him what we had found. His little budgerigar was flitting about the room and settled on Lord Moran's shoulder, then he moved on to John and looked as though he was going to peck his ear. So I put out my finger and the little bird hopped on to it. Winston chuckled so much that I don't think he paid any attention to what we were saying.

76ᵗʰ birthday.

Nov. 30ᵗʰ. 8.15 good action of bowels soft stool.

12.15 pm. visited by Lord Moran & Seddon. Comfortable though he looks weary. Sprius: no pain or old freeing on heavy palpation. May get up for lunch in Lady Churchill's room.

45° mattress rest has been made for his big bed. Installed in the evening: most successful.

Dec. 1ˢᵗ up for lunch & dinner, latter semi-dressed. up till 10.30 pm. cheerful.

Dec. 2ⁿᵈ.

29. Handwritten notes

<u>4.12.60.</u> A most disturbing development, a definite angular deformity at the cervico-thoracic junction which looked rather more like what one sees fairly often in old people. Had there been a second fracture? I telephoned Lord Moran in Stafford and then Golding.

The latter told me that with a man of Sir Winston's broad shoulders it was nearly impossible to take lateral tomographs, the only x-rays that would be of the slightest use. I told him that he had got to take the x-rays, even if his apparatus blew up. He spent a little time practising on someone with shoulders resembling Winston's and on the afternoon of December 5th we went by ambulance to Golding's rooms. By this time I was thoroughly sick of our being trailed by reporters, and I took a small suitcase with me containing what I thought was an appropriate disguise. Golding took some superb pictures and they showed an old lesion of the 4th to the 7th cervical vertebrae which were all fused. There was no change in the state of the 5th thoracic.

It must have been difficult to imagine the old and weighty patient as a young man, but when young and active he had played polo, fought in wars in Africa and been injured in various ways. As a boy Winston was involved in a chase with his younger brother and a cousin, which ended in a leap from a bridge to trees. Winston missed the trees and so fell nine metres; the branches mitigated his fall somewhat, but he probably damaged his spine at this time – a fact recognised by Seddon, who had read Churchill's account of his early life.[138]

After this episode in Campbell Golding's place I donned my disguise, a light raincoat, a soft hat, pulled a bit over one eye and I left the place with my hands in my pockets without a single one of the reporters recognising me. I left them to tackle Lord Moran who knew exactly how to deal with them.

The *Daily Telegraph* printed a photograph of the tall, elegant "Mr Yeoman and his physiotherapist". Seddon looked rather bent and untidy in the picture. The extrovert Karl Nissen said to him "Jim, did you see that picture in the paper?" Seddon managed to laugh at this. There was more laughter when the time came for the hospital Christmas variety show to be performed; it was interrupted with the words "We have just had a call from Mr Churchill's home. Would his

---

138 Winston Churchill, *My Early Life* (Fontana, 1959), pp. 37, 38.

physio go to see him?" – a joke that went down very well with the audience.

> 27.1.61 Last visit ... Nine weeks after the injury, Sir Winston was, in Lord Moran's view, back to where he had been before.

In May, Lord Moran consulted W Russell Brain, the neurologist, who had first seen Churchill as a patient in 1949.[139] He viewed the x-rays and also concluded that, as well as old injuries, Churchill had sustained a crush fracture that affected the 6 cervical root.[140]

On 31 January 1961, Seddon wrote from the RNOH to Churchill's secretary, Montague Browne, about the delicate matter of payment for his services. Montague Browne had been appointed as secretary by the prime minister, Harold Macmillan, to give Churchill the assistance that he very badly needed.

> Lady Churchill was good enough to speak to Lord Moran and you to my secretary about my fee for attending Sir Winston.
>
> Sir Winston returned to the House of Commons last Thursday. That I was able to help towards this is sufficient reward, and if he and Lady Churchill have no objection I would prefer to leave it that way.
>
> May I take this opportunity of thanking you most warmly for the many acts of kindness during what was, for a while, rather an anxious undertaking.
>
> Yours sincerely,
>
> Herbert Seddon[141]

Churchill's reply is equally flowery:

> My Dear Seddon
>
> Montague Browne has shown me your letter of January 31. Please allow me to express to you my gratitude for all your skill and care during my illness, and my warm thanks for the graceful terms in which you

---

139 Moran 1966.
140 W Russell Brain.
141 CHUR 2/530 A/32.

phrase your letter.

It was indeed fortunate for me that I should have been attended by you and I am well aware of the trouble you took.

I hope that you will accept a photograph and a copy of my biography of MARLBOROUGH which I have signed for you.

Yours very sincerely

WWSC[142]

Seddon wondered if he might comment on the book. He asked Montague Browne about this:

RNOH 6.2.61

My dear Montague Browne

You are a wise counsellor. Will you please read the enclosed letter. I have no means of knowing how Sir Winston would regard an expression of an opinion on the writing of history from someone who is no more than an enthusiastic dabbler. But he could not have sent me a more welcome gift, and that is why I have written rather more than a simple letter of thanks.

If you have any doubts send the letter back to me, if you please. I was greatly touched by your personal note: I too hope that we may meet again though I trust on a sunnier occasion.

Yours sincerely

HJ Seddon[143]

It seems that Browne's response was positive, since this letter was sent:

Dear Sir Winston

I am grateful to you and to Lady Churchill for your extremely kind letters. And may I say how delighted I am to have this excellent photograph and the signed volumes of your biography of MARLBOROUGH.

May I dilate a little on the last. I have not yet read all

---

142 CHUR 2/530 A/38, letter of 2 February 1961. ©Winston S. Churchill.
143 CHUR 2/530 A/35 and 34.

of your books – The River War was to have been the next – but of those I know MARLBOROUGH is my favourite. Other historians have busied themselves with this glorious period in our history, but I have not yet come across a picture of it that can compare with yours. And when the subject of a biography is a hero, and Marlborough was in all conscience, I applaud the writer who brings out the heroic lineaments; when this is done the faults, the human failings, are usually faithfully dealt with too. Two kindred examples, among many, come to mind, Carola Oman's NELSON and, more recently, Margery Perham's LUGARD. I detest works like Strachey's EMINENT VICTORIANS; and for that reason I am glad you dished Macaulay.

I hope you will forgive these elementary observations, but in sending me this biography, which I prize so highly, you have touched on one of my interests. The River War will have to wait and I must read MARLBOROUGH again.

I shall not forget the great kindness of Lady Churchill and of yourself that so greatly lightened Lord Moran's and my task.

                    Yours sincerely
                    HJ Seddon

Churchill was pleased with and interested in the letter. He and Lady Churchill left for Monte Carlo, where they stayed at the Hôtel de Paris. Churchill was on the whole well, but getting rather bored by June, when Seddon had occasion to write again to Montague Browne:

Campbell Gordon, the radiologist whose aid was indis-pensable when Sir Winston broke his spine (sorting out the old injury from the recent one was quite a difficult job technically) came to see me a day or two ago about another puzzling patient. At the end of our talk he asked me, with all the diffidence in the world, whether there would be any possibility of his having a photograph of

Sir Winston for his study.

I said I had no idea and that you were the only person who could tell him or me. But he was even hesitant about getting in touch with you himself; so I said I would do so knowing well that you would tell me straight if the answer was no.

I have just been in Greece giving some lectures for the British Council and there I met Professor Garofilides, a most exuberant man.

My best wishes to you.

Yours sincerely

H.J. Seddon[144]

The request was granted, and Sir Winston sent his very good wishes to Seddon.

In June 1962 Churchill was again in Monte Carlo, when he fell and broke his hip. At his request he was flown back to London, to the Middlesex Hospital, after being x-rayed and put in an extensive plaster. "He was cheerful and not distressed and in particular said he had no pain in the back".[145] He was operated on at 6 p.m. on 29 June 1962. OP Dinnick and DH Cope gave the anaesthetic. The fracture was reduced and Philip Newman inserted a plate and pin, assisted by Seddon who had had little recent practice in pinning hips. Churchill made a good recovery. Seddon wrote:

A personal note. During his stay in the Middlesex Sir Winston said that he found the evenings burdensome: would I come in at times and keep him company? I explained about having to work at Stanmore as well as in town, but said I would come in when I could. We agreed that I should come at coffee time and I would have my dinner first at one of the little restaurants in Soho. When I arrived the coffee, brandy and cigars appeared. Sir Winston poured the coffee himself and always asked whether I preferred white or brown sugar. Then the brandy. Incidentally (I have no idea what he

---

144 CHUR 2/530 A/35 and 34. Churchill knew Professor Theodore Garofilides.

145 M Gilbert, Winston S. Churchill: the official biography, London: Heinemann, 8 vols (1966–88), Vol. 8, p. 1334.

was like in his younger days) I have never met anyone who could make a modest dose of cognac last so long. The big ceremonial was choosing the cigar; about four boxes were placed on his bed tray. Each was opened and he pawed through the cigars to find one that was exactly right; he sniffed them, he rolled them between his fingers and listened to them. What good that did defeated me, because he was deafer than me. I think I smoked these great cigars on three evenings. Then I gave up; they were just too big, and I asked if I might light a pipe instead. He agreed but added – about the cigars – "you're still young: it's simply a matter of experience". Sometimes we talked. He waxed enthusiastic about Marrakesh and painting there. I said I had been once, and even done a little painting.

Even if they differed on tobacco, Seddon and Churchill had at least two things in common. Seddon had been completely deaf in his left ear for many years and for at least the last 20 years had worn a hearing aid in the right ear. During the bitter winter of 1963, when snow lay for three months, Seddon was prevented from gardening and so he had taken up painting in oils and with watercolours.

Newman and Seddon were consulted about the practical arrangements for Churchill's return home from hospital. Seddon arranged to visit 28 Hyde Park Gate on 28 July, but he perhaps had to cancel this or his next visit because Churchill sent a telegram on 1 August to say he was sorry Seddon was unwell. Seddon replied from Lake House on 2 August 1962:

Dear Sir Winston,
Thank you for your very kind message.
It is no more than a trifling upset. I think I should be back to full activity by the time you receive this note and I am looking forward to paying you a visit after lunch on Sunday. I shall be particularly interested to learn if you are finding yourself steadier and stronger on your feet.

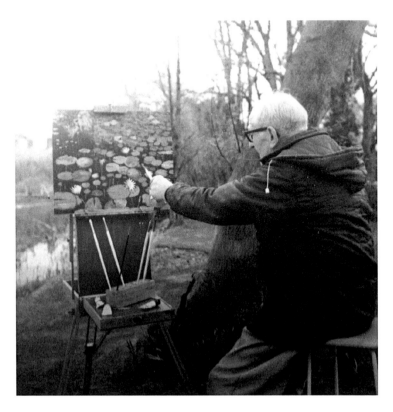

30. Seddon painting at Lake House

My Philip Yeoman is having a holiday with his young family, so I am rather busy. However, I hope I shall be able to come one evening next week – quite apart from official visits – at about the time when coffee is brought into your room. You make me so welcome.
Yours sincerely,
Herbert Seddon.[146]

Later that month Seddon wrote to Montague Browne (on 22 August, from Malcolm House, Batsford, Moreton-in-Marsh) that the instructions for a shallow bath that could easily be stepped into had been misunderstood and that the step that had been built beside the

---

146 CHUR1/62/27.

bath would, in fact, make it more difficult to get in. He added that he and Philip Newman were going to Copenhagen for a surgical meeting, but Philip Yeoman would be available if needed. He added that he would be in East Africa as a member of a commission from 14 September until about 12 October. Montague Browne replied:

> I am sorry there has been a misunderstanding about the step, but I think all is well: Sir Winston has declined to use it and has got in and out of his bath with considerable agility! He has also walked twice to the drawing room using your rail.

In lieu of fees for the care of Sir Winston, Seddon was given an inscribed silver swing-handled basket dated 1797, a box of 50 cigars and a letter of thanks. Mr Newman and Dr Golding were also given silver and cigars.

> 17th September, 1962
>
> My Dear Seddon,
> I think you know how grateful I am for all your devotion and skill, which has enabled me to regain my health. I will not therefore enlarge on them beyond saying that I shall always remember what you have done for me.
> I hope that you will accept these mementos of our association.
> Yours very sincerely,
> W.S.C.[147]

On receiving the parcel, Mary Seddon immediately wrote to Montague Browne to say that her husband was already in East Africa and that she was just leaving for Italy. She asked him to explain to Lady Churchill why the parcel would not be opened yet and that thanks would have to be deferred. Seddon was visiting East Africa as a member of the Committee on (East African) University Needs and Priorities. On his return he wrote:

---

147 CHUR1/62/118. © Winston S. Churchill.

Dear Sir Winston,

I have just returned from East Africa. You thank me most generously. May I, in reply, recall the words of a sixteenth century surgeon, Ambroise Paré, "Je le pausay, Dieu le guarit."

What a delight it is to possess such a superb piece of silver, with an inscription perfect in its simplicity. This is not for me alone, it is for my family.

And how kind of you to add a box of cigars: I have not yet finished my first supply!

In thanking you for these mementos may I also say how grateful I am to Lady Churchill for her patience and understanding, and to you, Sir Winston, for your kindness to Philip Newman and me – your faithful servants – , which made our anxiety easier to bear.

Yours sincerely
Herbert Seddon.[148]

Telegrams were exchanged on Sir Winston's 88th birthday:

Best wishes from two surgeons who hope in the words of the 51st Psalm that the bones which thou hast broken may rejoice.
Philip Newman and Herbert Seddon.

I am grateful to you for your telegram and thanks to you both. Psalm 73 verse 2 no longer applies.
Winston S. Churchill

The verse quoted is: "But as for me, my feet were almost gone; my steps had well nigh slipped."

Seddon was familiar with the bible. His childhood background was with the Plymouth Brethren, but he had never accepted this severe tradition of Christianity. In Stanmore he was an active parishioner at the Anglican church of St John. The rector, Stephen Skemp, suggested that he have some brief training and become a lay preacher when he retired. Seddon took up the suggestion eagerly and gave a meticulously prepared sermon about once a month. One

---

148 CHUR1/62/71.

Battle of Britain Sunday he was invited to give the sermon. It was a formal occasion in the presence of representatives of the RAF, the mayor and councillors, but he was aware of its comic potential: he was wearing his scarlet doctor's hood and blue reader's scarf over a white surplice. Before he began, he leaned over the pulpit and said "You probably wonder what I am doing here, looking like some decrepit Union Jack".

His work in the church was not trivial. For example, he initiated a series of visiting preachers for Lent that included up-and-coming churchmen like Runcie, the future Archbishop of Canterbury. Typically he made contact with him when he went one day to paint St Albans Abbey. Looking back to his time at school when he was persuaded to choose medicine as a career, Seddon wrote a pamphlet, *Fitness in Medicine*, to advise students who had decided to pursue medicine. It was published in May 1962 by the Christian Medical Fellowship.[149]

Seddon was asked to visit his famous patient at Chartwell at the end of August 1963. There is a footnote to the Churchill consultations, in the form of a note from a member of Churchill's staff, a year later. It reads: "I think this must be your lost pen? I am very sorry we did not find it before. Apparently it was in Sir Winston's study all the time, and lots of people looked at it and thought it belonged there!"[150] It did in fact belong to the absent-minded Professor Seddon.

January of the next year began with Seddon receiving a great accolade (Fig 25), a knighthood which was announced on 3 January 1964 in the New Year honours list. Among the congratulations came a telegram from Winston and Clementine. Seddon sent a handwritten reply:

RNOH
234 Great Portland Street
4th Jan. 1964

Dear Sir Winston

Your approbation means much to me, and I am very grateful to you and to Lady Churchill for your kind

---

149 Seddon 1962b.
150 CHUR 2/534 69 of 23 September 1963.

message of congratulation.
My best wishes to you both, and my thanks.
Yours sincerely
Herbert Seddon[151]

Back at the RNOH he was given a new nickname, 'Sherbert'! From the USA, Sally and Michael sent a telegram "Congratulations: early recognition of artistic genius" so Jim pasted the message under a photograph of a chimpanzee doing a painting.

That would have been the end of the story, except that in October 1965 Lady Churchill's arm was broken. The trauma was caused by a football hitting her and causing her to fall on her arm when she was walking in Hyde Park. Seddon was consulted and the news was widely reported, even in the Ellensburg *Daily Record* in faraway Washington State.

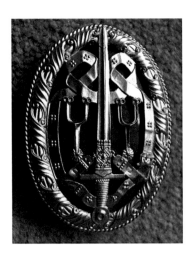

31. Emblem of a Knight, showing sword and spurs

151 The telegram from Winston and Clementine is CHUR 2/534/68. Seddon's reply is also in CHUR 2/534.

Chapter 14

Academic recognition, more medals and retirement

As a past president of the British Orthopaedic Association, Seddon was now an elder statesman of surgery, invited to chair committees, write and give lectures. In 1962 the University of Edinburgh awarded him the Lawrence Poole Prize, which was worth £60, a useful sum in those days. It also included a two-day visit to the Edinburgh Medical School and an invitation to lecture on the subject of disabling motor disease.

He still had day-to-day responsibility for the Institute of Orthopaedics and his work at the Royal National Orthopaedic Hospital, at Stanmore and Great Portland Street. The RNOH buildings at Stanmore were in need of modernisation, and plans had been made to build a new hospital in a horseshoe design. The work was started in 1962, but the only parts completed were two new operating theatres.

At the Royal College of Surgeons, Seddon delivered the fourth Ruscoe Clarke Memorial Lecture on 23 May 1963, taking as his subject Volkmann's ischaemia.[152] Alan Ruscoe Clarke established the reputation of the accident service in Birmingham, starting from the work done by him and his colleagues during the war. He was known for his communist beliefs at a time when the cold war was a major political concern; some people felt that Seddon showed unjustified bias against the Birmingham department.[153]

The year 1963 was one of dramatic events. It had started well, with Martin Luther King declaring against racial prejudice "I have a dream" but later that year the spy Kim Philby defected to the USSR, the Profumo affair erupted and in November President John F Kennedy was assassinated, to mention but a few of the disasters. That same year, Seddon gave the fourth Watson-Jones Lecture of the Royal College of Surgeons of England. He was becoming a more relaxed speaker and told several stories:

---

152 RCS Eng., 23 May 1963.
153 Seddon 1964.

For the first time in my life I find myself delivering an eponymous lecture in the presence of the eponym – only a shade less embarrassing than for a man having to deliver a lecture named after himself. This is what happened to Dr Wilder Penfield in Beirut in the spring of 1961; he felt, he said at the time, a little posthumous. I mention this, Mr President, simply as a suggestion for your consideration when choosing a later Watson-Jones lecturer.[154]

Another of the stories he told was about a singing Irishman and a surgical mistake Seddon had made. He could afford to reveal it now. The real subject of the lecture was nerve grafting,[155] a theme on which he again spoke at a conference in Brussels a few years later.[156] He acknowledged Don Brooks' work that had made nerve grafting "respectable" and he recorded the first clearly documented success from intercostal transfer to restore active flexion of the elbows, the operation performed with Yeoman.[157] Philip Yeoman's work was part of a PhD for the University of Cambridge.

Seddon had lectured in the Lebanon and demonstrated operations there, for example on post-polio cases and on peripheral nerves, when he had been assisting the Colonial Service. English was the language used. The Lebanon was at that time a wealthy country, where an extravagant lifestyle was enjoyed by the elite. Money was spent on shows with fantastic staging or could be gambled away in casinos, but for Seddon the spectacular scenery was a bigger attraction. In 1963, he had another invitation to visit the Lebanon, and this time Mary and Sally came too.

Sally and Jim started to climb one of the beautiful Lebanese mountains, which in winter are snow-covered while the coast is still

---

154 Wilder Penfield discovered much about brain function. Among his many honours over a long life – he was 70 at the time of the Beirut lecture– was the Order of Merit. He came to Oxford in 1914 as a Rhodes Scholar at Merton College, where he was influenced by Charles Sherrington and Osler, and became friends with 'wee Georgie' Riddoch. He became a neurosurgeon, learning from Harvey Cushing in Boston, then spent most of his career in Montreal. His autobiography, No Man Alone, was published in 1977, a year after his death.

155 Seddon 1963.

156 Seddon 1967.

157 Birch, Bonney and Wynn Parry 1998.

warm. Towards the top, Jim became breathless and unable to continue. Sally was unsure what to do but in the end left Jim to rest while she made it to the summit, the highest in the region. They decided to tell Mary nothing of this worrying incident.

He spoke on Volkmann's ischaemic contracture at the 1963 conference of the Middle East Medical Assembly (MEMA), again hosted by the American University of Beirut.[158] The Faculty Bulletin reported that "Prof. Herbert J. Seddon, Director of Studies at the Institute of Orthopaedics at the University of London … is one of the greatest living orthopaedic surgeons of the world. Last year he nailed the hip of Sir Winston Churchill and now Churchill is walking. He has previously attended a MEMA meeting".[159] On this visit he also presented orthopaedic problem cases at a clinical conference.

From 1967 to 1974 he continued to work for a month at a time in the Lebanon as a Consulting Orthopaedic Surgeon to the Lebanese Army, making fifteen trips in all. Later this work continued with Philip Yeoman and Don Brooks. The anaesthetist Denis O'Donaghue went too. Seddon was highly respected in the Lebanon and honoured by that country. He was made an officer of the National Order of the Cedar in 1966 (an award created at the end of 1936) and was awarded Order of Merit, first class, Lebanon in 1974. He also held honorary degrees from the University of Grenoble and the Royal University of Malta. The University of Glasgow gave him an honorary LlD in 1965.

The Second Hand Club was, despite its delightful name, nothing to do with charity shops, but quite a learned group. In 1964 Seddon addressed a joint meeting between them and the Scandinavian Club for the Surgery of the Hand. He presented a paper on Volkmann's ischaemia[160] that was to be published in the *British Medical Journal*.

---

158 3rd MEMA Report, III-I-5 (May 1963).
159 *American University of Beirut Faculty Bulletin*, 27 April 1963, pp. 1–2. Seddon also spoke at MEMA's 1961 meeting.
160 Report, *JBJS*, **46B** 359. For the *BMJ* publication, see Seddon 1964.

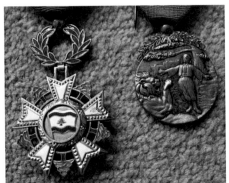

Fig 32. Lebanese honours

Seddon still enjoyed going abroad and in April of that year he went to Greece with the Orthopaedic Travelling Club (two years earlier he had been to Llandudno with them) for a meeting in Athens organised jointly with the Hellenic Orthopaedic Society. Talking about paralysis of muscles around the hip joint, he said there were four problems: paralysis, contracture, subluxation and dipping gait. He could cite a hundred cases and their treatment that he had reviewed.[161] He and DW Parsons from the Institute of Orthopaedics published a joint paper three years later on 'The results of operations for disorders of the hip caused by poliomyelitis'.[162]

Although orthopaedics was taught at the institute in Great Portland Street and though the institute had joined the Postgraduate Medical Federation founded by the University of London, it had no other academic status. This was remedied in 1965 when a personal chair in orthopaedic surgery was created for Seddon as part of the University of London. It was supported by a grant of £100,000 from the National Fund for Research into Poliomyelitis and Other Crippling Diseases (now the charity Action Medical Research). The charity's report, in Appendix 41, stated that "this chair ... will bring London to a position level with Oxford, Liverpool, Manchester, Edinburgh and Glasgow". Thus, after being Director of the Institute of Orthopaedics for eighteen years, Seddon at last regained the title of professor that he had lost when he left Oxford; however, only two years after becoming professor he reached the retirement age of 65.

The registrar he invited to be his first assistant and senior

---

161 Report of the British Orthopaedic Travelling Club', *JBJS*, **31B** 802.
162 Parsons and Seddon 1968.

lecturer on the professorial unit was Alan Lettin, an outspoken and bright young surgeon who had grown up in the east end of London. He first came to the RNOH to work under Philip Newman, who was trying out a number of new prostheses for hip, knee and shoulder, and Charles Manning, who ran the scoliosis unit. When promoted to registrar, Alan Lettin worked with different consultants, changing every six months as was the norm.

Lettin later wrote his autobiography under the title *Was it something I said?* Seddon did sometimes find it rather difficult working with someone who was not so deferential as was usual and who insisted on having the last word. When Lettin asked for a reference, Seddon mentioned that he might be awkward to get on with and this frankness lost Lettin his first application for a consultant post.

When Seddon became professor, he diminished his operating list at Stanmore; a typical operating list was now only one to four cases, but some were very long and intricate. This gave him time to arrange meetings on special subjects at Stanmore. As professor, he supervised research and continued to be published.[163] Some of his time was spent in lecturing but, as he freely admitted, he was not a very exciting lecturer and his lectures were poorly attended. There was only one thing to be done.

He sought the assistance of Derek Sayer, a technician working on the problems of arthritis. At the next lecture, the students were jolted awake by a slide showing a pretty young woman in a bathing costume. Seddon pretended to be amazed, indignant and quite ignorant of how such a slide could have got in among his. Students laughed and spread the word. More students came to the next lecture and somehow yet another saucy slide appeared during the lecture, again to Seddon's apparent confusion. The schoolboy joke continued and the lectures became very popular. When Seddon retired he gave his microscope to Derek Sayer.

Another view comes from a colleague who heard one of his last lectures at the hospital and remembered the frailty that made him apologise for remaining seated, but also the riveted attention of the audience as he developed his theme so quietly, logically and powerfully.

---

163 Leffert and Seddon 1965; Howse and Seddon 1966.

The Orthopaedic Section of the Royal Society of Medicine conferred honorary membership on Seddon and Merle d'Aubigné at the end of 1965, for which they were given a diploma in March 1966. Worcester College, Oxford gave him an honorary fellowship. Seddon retired in 1967 from his post at RNOH and the Institute, and became an honorary consulting surgeon there. When he retired from that post in 1975, the RNOH and Institute presented him with a silver salver. Professor Geoffrey Burwell succeeded Seddon in 1967. He brought a fresh vision to the RNOH and did much to modernise the Institute of Orthopaedics. He was particularly interested in bone transplantation.

A dinner was held to mark the retirement of Seddon and AT Fripp, who had been the Dean of the Institute for two years. Fripp was presented with a deep freeze for his Sussex cottage. Hugh Micklem, son of one of the members of the hospital board, was an artist and he presented Sir Herbert with a portrait of himself; a second one was given to the hospital. It now hangs in the RNOH at Stanmore.

The RNOH created a silver medal called the H Jackson Burrows Medal, which it awarded in 1971 to Sir Harry Platt 'for meritorious academic achievement'. In 1975 it was awarded to Sir Herbert Seddon.

Another silver medal, named the Seddon Medal, was endowed by The Governors and Friends of the Royal National Orthopaedic Hospital together with £300 to be awarded by the hospital and institute in alternate years. Its intention was "to recognise outstanding clinical research within the scope of the holder of a clinical post at the Hospital below the grade of consultant". It was awarded to JR Condon in 1970 for work done the previous year on rickets and osteomalacia.

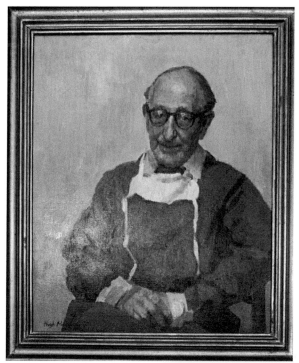

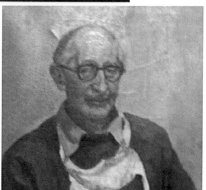

33. The painting of Sir Herbert Seddon by Hugh Micklem,
given to him, and detail of the RNOH portrait

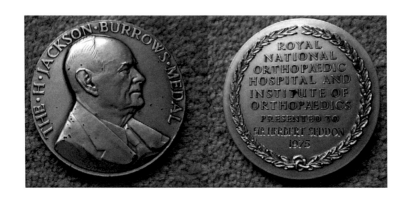

34. The RNOH Jackson Burrows Medal
presented in 1975

Chapter 15

The prodigal son is brought to book

When Seddon decided to retire from the professorship and his post as director of the institute, he at last felt confident of finding some time for writing. It was nearly 25 years since he had agreed to write a book for E & S Livingstone, and Charles Macmillan had probably given up hope of ever seeing a typescript, especially as Seddon had chosen another publisher for an earlier book. So his joy was all the greater when news did arrive. On 25 April 1966 the Professor of Orthopaedics Sir Herbert Seddon, CMG, DM, FRCS wrote thus to his old friend:

> Dear Charles
> You may recall that about twenty years ago I promised to write a book on nerve injuries.
> Because I have been so busy here, because I have spent a good deal of time stirring up orthopaedics in Africa and because I have not got the drive of Reginald Watson-Jones I have been a defaulter. At long last I hope to keep this promise.
> Some time when you are in London we ought, perhaps, to have a word about this business. You might feel like dining with me at the Athenaeum; the prodigal son would do his best to lay on a very modest fatted calf.
> Yours sincerely,
> Herbert Seddon.

Charles Macmillan seized the day and replied: "What a delightful letter to receive, such as the one you have written to me of 25th April. Nothing could give me greater pleasure than the prospect of having your name in our list of authors." He suggested dates when he would be in London and concluded "Whatever you desire, you may be sure that I will be delighted to fall in with your wishes.

You have certainly cheered me up immensely and the prospect of having a book from you thrills me."

In August 1966, Seddon was considering what to include in his book and what could usefully be re-used, as he explained to Macmillan: "In the J.B.J.S. 1963 45B, 447 is a paper of mine on nerve grafting. It was right up-to-date at the time and almost all of the illustrations would be useful for the book. If you still have the blocks it would be a nice economy to hang on to them." [They were indeed still available.] He was feeling optimistic: "The work is progressing and I am shortly taking two weeks off to devote the whole of my time to it. Yours ever, Herbert Seddon."

The next query he had for Macmillan was about illustrations:

> I have been giving earnest thought to the diagrams that will be necessary to illustrate nerve degeneration and regeneration. Diagrams are essential; photographs are no good.
>
> I enclose a copy of some diagrams that appeared in a very good book on histology by Ham of Toronto. The drawing is not bad though it could be better. What stands out a mile is that in order to make these drawings intelligible it is essential to use block colour and on the attached rough sketch I have tried to indicate what I mean. Three colours would do nicely and what I want to ask you is whether if one used, say, blue and yellow the combination of the two would give you a third colour, green, as I have shown. This would reduce cost.
>
> For these diagrams to be done correctly a great deal of specialised knowledge is necessary and for this reason I think it would save an immense amount of trouble if I did them myself. You must not judge of my efforts from this sketch which I dashed off in twenty minutes. I would use Indian ink, not marking ink.

Macmillan was on holiday so another director, James Parker, replied:

> Regarding the diagrams in which you wish to use flat
> colour, there should be no difficulty in obtaining further
> colours from the three primaries. The most economical
> way is to have the drawings made completely separated
> for colour. I would suggest that you make drawings two
> times the size required in the final book.

The publisher preferred to employ a professional artist called Robin Callender: "Our artist has made a copy from your drawing, showing the procedure he uses in making colour separations of the type suitable for your book. The separations for the colour are done on a material called Kodatrace." This was a type of film like Astrafoil, a transparent cover stable under varying atmospheric conditions which Parker recommended for adding colour layers to a line drawing.

> I would suggest 6⅞ × 9¾ for the size of page, which is
> approximately the same as the specimen from Ham's
> book. I enclose a specimen page which we prepared for
> a book by Kunkler & Rains and you may find this
> useful for making up the types to be used in your
> manuscript.

Seddon planned to attend the BOA meeting in Edinburgh in late September 1966 but he had to miss a splendid dinner there: "I am sorry about this, because your hospitality is wonderful and I know of no more pleasant place for a dinner than the College of Surgeons in Edinburgh". Mary travelled with him. At the meeting he joined in the discussion about the use of Millipore to wrap nerves before secondary surgery.[164]

He wrote to Macmillan:

> "I have been thinking again and very hard about the
> half-tone illustrations on shiny paper being interleaved
> with the letterpress on matt paper and I very much fear
> we shall find ourselves obliged to follow the prevailing
> fashion of shiny paper from start to finish. I hope you
> have had a good holiday. I look forward to mine, but it

---

164 *JBJS*, **49B**, 186. 1967.

does not come until November."

He pressed on with the work.

Dear Charles,

At this stage in the preparation of the book I am finding it expedient to devote a good deal and time and effort to the illustrations and by the New Year there will be a mass of stuff that I should discuss with Robin Callander. Am I at liberty to write to him direct and make my own arrangements? Is he aware of what is afoot?

I expect to be in Edinburgh in February 1967 to give a lecture at the College and I could take this opportunity of having a session with Callander; it might be better for me to go to Glasgow, rather than ask him to come over to Edinburgh because he may have stuff in his studio that would give me bright ideas about how this or that should be presented.

I now have a few questions for you.

1. Would you please look at the enclosed proofs which I have had in my files for twenty years. In one chapter there will be a very considerable number of diagrams showing areas of sensory loss and areas (unshaded) where there is no sweating. I am sure that diagrams are better than HT, but you will note that there are several methods of shading. Which do you favour?

2. Whitley is producing some glorious photographs. What I would like to know is whether you would like the original negatives sent with the prints. [In the margin of the letter: No]

3. If an illustration appears on, say, page 30 and there is an important reference to it on page 216 does it add very greatly to the expense if the illustration is repeated? You may say that it is expensive for HT but not for line drawing. I would welcome your guidance.

4. I wonder if you still have the blocks, in particular the colour blocks for Figures 1 and 2 of my article in the J.B.J.S. 1956 38B, 152. Some of them would be most useful. [Marginal note: Blocks destroyed.]

> My best wishes to you.
> Yours ever,
> Herbert Seddon.

A reply came on 21 September 1966 from James Parker, because Charles Macmillan was attending the Frankfurt Book Fair, and a further reply from Macmillan on 28 October 1966. Even at Christmas he was giving time to the book.

> 28th December, 1966
>
> Dear Charles,
> I have been immensely impressed with the line drawings that are appearing in Fripp & Shaw's book on club foot. Could you spare me a proof sheet on any of these? I want to make use of this.
> Yours sincerely
> Herbert Seddon.

Two and a half months later the pace on the book had slowed, as he explained to Macmillan:

> I am struggling with my writing, but it will not go really well until I retire from my appointment here.
> Robin Callander has already done some illustrations for me and they exceed my expectations. I am very grateful to you for putting me in touch with him.
> I heard a little while ago that you yourself will shortly be retiring from Livingstone's; this is the gloomiest news of the year and however able your successor I shall find it difficult to talk as freely with him as I can do with you.
> Yours sincerely,
> Herbert Seddon

Macmillan received the letter when he returned from holiday in Ireland:

> Let me try and clear away your gloom. Although I am changing labels and dropping the title of Managing Director, I still hope to be about the office and to attend personally to your book to see it safely through the press. I am being relieved of the daily running of the business and I intend to devote more time to our authors and journals.
> Be assured that I am looking forward to dealing with your book with great enthusiasm.
> With kindest regards

On Tuesday 6 June 1967, a dinner was held in honour of Charles Macmillan and his fellow directors James Parker and EA Scott at the Adam Rooms of the George Hotel in Edinburgh. They were expecting 96 guests, many of whom had spent their working lives in this firm.

E & S Livingstone was absorbed into the Pearson Group, who already owned J & A Churchill, and so the imprint Churchill Livingstone was born in 1972. It was under this mark that Herbert Seddon's book was finally published. Longman & Green was added to the group, bringing together an impressive list of prestigious medical titles. Inevitably the nature of the company changed once it was part of a corporate empire. The Longman history, *At the Sign of the Ship* by Philip Wallis, records that changes were to be expected:

> The Ship that Hitler's bombs burned down,
> In Clifford Street gained fresh renown;
> It anchors now near Grosvenor Square,
> And this is just its Chairman's prayer –
> May Ship and Swan, and all the crew
> Accomplish what they try to do.
> May Grosvenor Street a haven prove
> Till growth doth force another move.

Churchill Livingstone adopted the Longman ship as its badge.

In November 1968 the Macmillans moved house, from 19 Wilton Road in the Newington area of Edinburgh to Braid Farm Road, south of Morningside.

1st January 1968

Dear Charles,

I am extremely grateful to you for sending me a presentation copy of Jip's splendid monograph on scoliosis which looks like being a winner. I suspect it is to some extent a carrot for the donkey, to make me go a little faster. I will take the hint.

Yours sincerely,

HJS

No doubt I shall be seeing you on January 19th and I look forward to it.

After typing the letter, Seddon added a note in ink: "No I shall not be there and thank you too for the calendar, a great favourite with my wife."

13th January 1968

Dear Charles,

Although the work on the book is not going quite as fast as either of us would like the pace will quicken very soon now and I hope I can go as fast as I did during the summer months.

I should be grateful for your advice about a small but delicate matter. The great Swiss drug firm, Sandoz, has asked me to write two thousand words for them about nerve injuries. They run a small journal called Triangle which has a wide circulation in I don't know how many languages and the contributors have to be four or five star people. I have written a very simple outline of advances in nerve repair and when I came to choose illustrations I could not help thinking of those I had already assembled (the illustrations for the book are pretty well complete); there are four, a very small part of the total number, and I myself would willingly let

Sandoz have them. But they are yours just as much as mine and the position is slightly different from taking an illustration from a book or journal that has already been published.

What do we do? My own feeling is that this article, with its extremely wide circulation, will be a very useful harbinger.

I should also like to have your permission to reproduce Figure 7 in the Journal, 1963, 45, 452.

Best wishes to you
        Yours ever
           Jim Seddon.

CM/MH   16th January, 1968.
I happened to call in at the Office before I left for London and found your letter of 13th January waiting for my attention. I am, therefore, replying to it from the big city.

I was delighted to know that you are making excellent progress with your important book and that you hope to make even greater progress during the summer months.

There is no problem about doing the article for Sandoz. I know the firm very well and I even know their Journal and I agree with you that they always try and get outstanding authorities to write for them. Nothing but good can come from your little article and if we wanted to get an advance free advertisement then may I suggest that you add a footnote to your article which could be couched as follows:

By courtesy of my publishers the illustrations are from my forthcoming book on "Peripheral Nerve Injuries" to be published shortly by E. & S. Livingstone Ltd.

You can alter the phraseology any way you wish but I do think it is important to mention your book and the publishers. This will do a lot of good I feel sure.

You certainly have my permission to reproduce Figure 7 in the Journal, 1963, 45, 452. If you would like the illustration itself I could send this on when I get back next week, but probably the original will be good enough for your purpose.

Yours sincerely,
Charles Macmillan

A month later, Seddon was giving the Lady Jones lecture at the University of Liverpool, named in honour of Robert Jones' wife.[165] He spoke of invention, research and wives. He mentioned the equanimity and good domestic management of Lady Jones that had contributed to "the happiness and to the success, in the best sense, of the greatest surgeon that Liverpool has known". By implication, Seddon did not expect wives to have careers outside the home. Certainly that had been the case in his marriage. Ever supportive of her husband, Mary typed the manuscript of Jim's book.

20th January, 1969

Dear Charles

You will not have received the letter I sent you to thank you for that lovely Scotsman calendar because it has been destroyed by fire at the post office; vandalism, we think.

The calendar this year is better than ever before, both in the shape and their use of colour. My wife and I are most grateful to you.

I have just received a copy of Sunderland's colossal book for review. I don't think I shall be able to read all of the 1,100 pages; this would interfere very seriously with my own work on a book on nerve injuries. What I am doing is, of course, entirely different; it will be a surgical text-book of modest proportions, lots of good illustrations and data based on an analysis of some 2,300 case histories.

I am painfully aware that the work is not going as fast as you would wish, but I think that at the finish you will be satisfied.

Alas I cannot come to the dinner next Friday; I do hope that I may have the pleasure of meeting you some other time when you are in London.

---

165 *JBJS*, **50B**, (1068) 428.

Seddon did find time to review Sunderland's book for the *Journal of Bone and Joint Surgery* and thought it patchy.[166] It had a foreword by Sir Frances Walsh, of whom Seddon says: "after reproving – more in sorrow than in anger – the wayward anatomists who forsake honest morphology he warmly commends Professor Sunderland's excursion into the clinical field. This is most encouraging because I can hardly be alone in having special admiration for that little band of anatomists – Huber, Stopford, Woollard, JZ Young, Weddell and most of all Sunderland who have interested themselves in disorders of the peripheral nerves and placed clinicians so much in their debt." In a letter to Macmillan, Seddon acknowledges that:

> No one in the world has written so much on the anatomy of the peripheral nerves as Professor Sutherland in Melbourne and I am not in the least surprised that his book runs to 75 chapters. On certain matters I shall be quoting him quite extensively, but he will not have a great deal to offer on the clinical side and there will, as you say, be little overlap between his book and mine.

> 9th July 1969
> 47 Braid Farm Road
> Edinburgh 10
> Tel. 031 447 7417

Dear Sir Herbert,
    I was delighted to get your letter of 26th June 1969. I go into the office only occasionally as I have terminated my association with the firm after giving them a full fifty years of service.
    It so happens that I will be in London on 24th of July. The officials in Bracken House are putting on a dinner in my honour and they are bidding me a 'fond farewell'. If we could meet for a light lunch I should be very happy indeed and if this date is suitable let me know.

---

166 Seddon 1969.

May I say how delighted I am that you are making some progress with the book on Nerve Injuries – I know it will be a classic. I am glad that even although your progress is not as swift as you would like, sometimes quiet patient work produces startling results.

I am looking forward to having a chat with you if it can be arranged to meet you for lunch on Thursday 24th July 1969.

Yours sincerely

Seddon gave Charles Macmillan a painting of Invercauld House, a grand mansion near Braemar in Scotland.

14th August 1969

Dear Charles,

I promised to let you have some news about what I have been doing about the book on nerve injuries.

During the period 1940–1945 I collected the records of some 2,500 patients and they are the most complete documents of their kind in existence. I had all the important information abstracted from these records, put on cards and then transferred to punched cards to be put through a sorter-counter. This took 18 months; I checked every card myself and the cost was £1,000, which I am happy to say has not come out of your pocket or mine. The point of all this is that the book is written on first-hand information about a very considerable number of patients; in only a few instances has it been necessary to draw on the work of others though, of course, reference is made to conclusions reached by other surgeons.

I am deliberately over-illustrating. I know how expensive half-tones are, colour still more so, but it is much better to knock things out than to put them in at the last minute. When the time comes I shall want one of the experts in Livingstone's, in collaboration with me, to do some pretty ruthless cutting of illustrations.* We don't want to make the book prohibitively

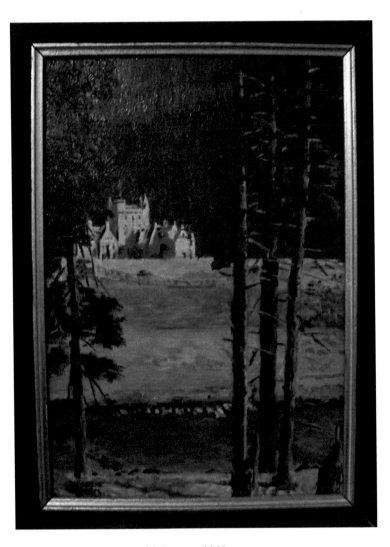

35. Invercauld House

expensive; I read those rather damning articles in the B.M.J. three weeks ago.

Each chapter is being read by a very knowledgeable person and you will be pleased to hear that Mr. Crawford Adams has been good enough to undertake the major part of the reading. He really is a superb editor.

There are 16 chapters of which 10 are completed. Theoretically I ought now to be able to go quite fast because the material is assembled. But I find that I am always having to go back to the sorter-counter machine to get answers to questions that arise in the course of the writing. Thus, I am reluctant to give you a date for the completion of the manuscript, but I hope that I shall not be trying Livingstone's patience for much longer.

Yours sincerely,

Herbert Seddon.

*This will not apply to any of the illustrations that Robert Callander has made: they are all essential.

The footnote to this letter was handwritten by Seddon.

Charles Macmillan was honoured with an OBE in 1970 for services to exports, in recognition of his contribution to medical publishing. His family saw him receive the award and celebrated afterwards. The final stages of Seddon's book were handled by Henderson, the new Managing Director, and others at Churchill Livingstone.

25th June 1970.

Dear Mr. Henderson,

The book on nerve injuries is almost finished.

My chief reader – I have roped in three other people for rather special chapters – is Mr. Crawford Adams.[167] You will agree that one could not have a better person; I think he is superb. A few nights ago he dined with me so that we could talk about the book, and he suggested that I should start feeding chapters in to you. However, before that begins I think we ought to meet. There are a

---

167 The author of 'Outline of Fractures, including Joint Injuries' reviewed by Seddon 1957c.

number of points that we should discuss and, in particular, the illustrations. I have deliberately over-illustrated because it is much easier to knock out illustrations than to add to their number. I have prepared a schedule, now almost complete, which is divided into three parts; diagrams, half-tone photographs, and colour ... all that you would need to do is say what number is reasonable. We don't want to price the book out of the market because of the high cost of illustration ...

There are a number of other minor matters that we might talk over. Although I have done a great deal of medical writing I am not at all informed about the technique of getting a book published; I have had only two experiences of this, both of them rather a long time ago.

I am not going to be away except for a function in Manchester that I must attend on July 9. If by some remote chance you yourself happened to be in Manchester then I would prolong my stay, spending the night there, and meet you. But my expectation is that it would be more convenient for you – as it would be for me – if we met on the occasion of one of your visits to London.

As Henderson was on holiday, he sent a memo on 3 July 1970 to the production director, AD Lewis, suggesting he went to London to give guidance on the illustrations. Seddon replied with suggested dates and instructions (numbered 1 to 7) how to get to Stanmore. He would meet Lewis at the station, give him shaving, bath facilities and breakfast at the house, and arrange a hire car to take him to the airport. Finally, and almost reluctantly, he wrote "if you wish to take away, say, ten chapters of MSS, I would have them ready for you in a rather shabby old bag." (Mary had been busy typing the manuscript but two and a half chapters were still incomplete.) Lewis declined breakfast but planned to take away as much of the manuscript as possible.

Surgical Disorders of the Peripheral Nerves by Sir Herbert Seddon was published in 1972. It contained 352 pages and 325 illustrations, almost one per page, and the price was £8. Seddon dedicated his book to the memory of Hugh Cairns and George Riddoch, two men who had been so instrumental in organising the treatment of nerve injuries during the Second World War. The book had a long author index, subject index and copious references. Churchill Livingstone recorded initial stock as 2,516 copies. More than 1,500 copies were sold in the year 1972–3 and over 600 the next year. In the following three years, sales dwindled to a few hundred a year, still a respectable figure for such a book.

Seddon had some criticisms of his own work and was a sharp critic of others. Shortly before his own book was reviewed in the *British Medical Journal*, he reviewed *Injuries to the Major Branches of Peripheral Nerves of the Forearm* by Morton Spinner, published by WB Saunders.[168] "The result is a mass of somewhat indigestible information" he growled, and he criticised the poor photographs of dissections. However, he admitted it was a most valuable work of reference. In the concluding words of his own book he criticised himself, regretting the lack of controlled clinical trials in his own work. But, he added, if such clinical trials were undertaken,

> two heads are not better than one ... as the single assessor, being human, is prone to err, but if he has any qualification for the job the errors will be small and *almost always in the same direction*. Thus such error as there is will have the same incidence in both groups of cases ... Forthright dogmatism is better than conclusions propped up by shaky statistics. To this sharp observation I add my regrets that I did not learn these lessons until late in my career as a surgeon.

Reviews appear quite slowly after a book is published.[169] At the Churchill Livingstone office, reviews of *Surgical Disorders of the Peripheral Nerves* were pasted on to the back of old E & S Livingstone notepaper and posted out to Seddon. The first review came from The Lancet and began "here is a monograph which is as near perfect as any can be". Even so, it suggested that "A section on medicolegal assessment of nerve lesions would have been useful".

---

168 Seddon 1972a.

Ruth Bowden who had worked with Seddon in Oxford was full of praise for his book:

> It is a beautifully illustrated, lucid, and remarkably brief – but closely reasoned – account of the many problems of diagnosis and treatment of surgical peripheral nerve disorders … It is a distillate of years of experience and the apologia pro vita sua of a surgeon who is a scholar and craftsman; a clinician who treats the whole patient.

Did she have any criticisms? Well, she would have liked some more microscopic pictures of healthy nerves and there were a few omissions. He had not mentioned the 1966 Ciba Foundation Symposium on 'Touch, heat and pain' or Professor David Sinclair's review *Cutaneous Sensation* (OUP 1967). She quibbled with the title, which she thought might put people off, but nonetheless

> Those who have enjoyed the stimulus and rigours of training by Sir Herbert will rejoice to see this distillate of clinical work, judgement and courage. As always, he pays the most generous tribute to his senior and junior colleagues who enriched his experience and made this book possible. The factual content and elegant brevity of the prose and the beautiful type and illustrations make the price reasonable.

It was reviewed far and wide. A review in the South African Medical Journal stated that

---

169 Book reviews of the 1st edition were published during 1972 in: *The Lancet* (8 April) with price given as £8, in USA Williams & Wilkins $25.60; *BMJ* (2 July), Vol. 3, p. 596, reviewer Ruth E Bowden; *Journal of the Irish Colleges of Physicians and Surgeons* (July); *British Journal of Surgery* (September), Vol. 59, p. 749; *British Journal of Hospital Medicine* (October), reviewer TT King; *Journal of Bone and Joint Surgery*, Vol. 54B (November), reviewer James Ellis; *Medical Journal of Australia* (October); Brain (October), reviewer CP Symonds; *Developmental Medicine and Child Neurology*, reviewer JF Shaw; *Journal of Neurology, Neurosurgery and Psychiatry* (December), reviewer AJ Simpson; *South African Medical Journal* (2 December), reviewer TS; and in 1974 in the *Postgraduate Medical Journal*, Vol. 50, No. 590, giving the price as £8.

This book is written in a delightfully modest and yet authoritative style. The author, long in the forefront of experimental and practical work on the subject, reviews the type of nerve injuries comprehensively ... this book should be at the bedside of every casualty officer and of every surgeon who is responsible for the management of Trauma.[170]

Both author and publisher must have felt very satisfied with the book that had been proposed so many years before and that was nearly never written.

Continued demand for *Disorders of the Peripheral Nerves* and changes in surgical techniques made a second edition imperative. As Seddon wrote in the preface, "It is becoming almost indecent not to use an operating microscope, and epineural suture is becoming obsolete". In the new edition there were also better micrographs provided by Professor PK Thomas.

The second edition of *Disorders of the Peripheral Nerves* was published in 1975. It was bound in black cloth with gilt lettering for the title, and had a blue dust cover. TA Constable in Edinburgh printed about a thousand copies of 346 pages each, and it remained in the Churchill Livingstone catalogue until 1988, when it was priced at £40. It was also translated into Japanese. Naoichi Tsuyama, who had been a British Council scholar in 1955–6 at the RNOH and who became Professor of Orthopaedic Surgery at the University of Tokyo, wrote to Seddon in perfect English that the book was"so welcomed by the orthopaedic surgeons in Japan".

New reviews appeared.[171] One reviewer, JA Simpson, writing

---

170 *South African Medical Journal/S.A. Mediese Tydskrif* (2 December 1972), p. 1912.
171 Reviews of the 2nd edition appeared in *British Book News* (November 1975); *Journal of Neurology, Neurosurgery and Psychiatry* (April 1976), reviewer AJ Simpson; JBJS (May 1976), reviewer AHG Murley; *Canadian Journal of Surgery*, Vol. 19 (July 1976), p. 369, reviewer JK Terzis, Dalhousie University, Halifax, NS, with price given as $43.25; *Orthopaedic Review*, Vol. 5, No. 7 (July 1976); Injury, Vol. 8, No. 1 (August 1976), reviewer TR Fisher; *Western Journal of Medicine* [USA] (August 1977), reviewer WE Stern, Dept of Surgery, University of California, LA Center for Health Sciences, price given as $39.50; *International Surgery* [USA], Vol. 19 (July or September 1976), p. 369, reviewer Roy Selby Jr, Lombard, Illinois; *Military Medicine* [USA] (1976), reviewer GE Omer.   197

for *Journal of Neurology, Neurosurgery and Psychiatry*, was aware of omissions and dared to be a little critical, although still full of praise.

A second edition in three years is sufficient testimony to the value of this outstanding book which is an essential work of reference for all who have to deal with peripheral nerve injuries. The revision includes more modern methods of electrodiagnosis but omits important data on the use of conduction studies for prognosis and monitoring of recovery, and of electromyography in detecting anomalous innervation, trick movements and aberrant regeneration. Modern immunology is just beginning to influence the use of homografts.

The age of transplant surgery was dawning and could only be successful with new discoveries in chemotherapy.

Entrapment syndromes receive a wider coverage but important 'medical' causes are omitted. The new knowledge of tourniquet paralysis receives only a passing reference. These points may indicate the desirability of greater co-operation between orthopaedic surgeon, physician and clinical physiologist to increase diagnostic precision. For the management of nerve injuries there is no better guide than this splendid book, because the author has the courage to describe his own doubts or occasional errors, so that this is more than a survey of recent publications. It is the recorded experience of the most distinguished surgeon in this field.

Other reviewers also pointed out omissions. For example, JK Terzis of Dalhousie University, Halifax, Nova Scotia, remarked in the *Canadian Journal of Surgery* that recent advances in clinical neurophysiology, microsurgical techniques and perineural repairs were alluded to in the preface but not described in the text "the section on operative treatment is therefore somewhat out of date".

Seddon was asked to review a book from Belgium, *New Developments on Myography and Clinical Neurophysiology*, edited by John E Desmedt. It was over thirty years since Seddon had worked with scientists in Oxford and his comment on this massive work of reference was that the subject was "now a gigantic industry".[172] In fact he compared its length, 2,000 pages, with that of the *New English Bible* (1,800 pages, minus Apocrypha). A bible and concordance were probably sitting on his desk ready to help him prepare something he would say as lay preacher at St John's. Sally remembers St Luke, patron saint of doctors and artists, coming into these sermons quite frequently. To encourage the reader of Desmedt's book he writes that "In places there is some sedate humour" and tantalisingly refers to an "account of myotonic goats".

---

172 *JBJS*, 1974.

Chapter 16

Epilogue

It is time to take look back on thirty years of work in this specialist field of peripheral nerve injuries, and where better to look than the meeting held in Paris by the Group d'Etude de la Main (GEM) in 1969. A book based on the papers presented at that meeting was published in French in 1972, as No. 2 in the GEM Monographs series, edited by Jacques Michon and Erik Moberg. The English translation (which Professor Moberg supervised) was the work of GEM and the Committee on Nerve Injuries under the direction of Seddon, and was published by Churchill Livingstone in 1975 as *Traumatic nerve lesions of the upper limb*.

It was probably Seddon who suggested to Macmillan that Churchill Livingstone might publish the work of GEM. This volume appeared in the same year as the second edition of Seddon's textbook, whose dust cover advertised the GEM book. The French orthopaedic surgeon Professor Robert Merle d'Aubigné wrote the preface to *Traumatic nerve lesions of the upper limb*, from which I quote:

> It was only during the Second World War that definite progress was made and principally in England by the concentration of these specific injuries within centres where a concerted effort could be made towards developing methods of clinical examination and investigation, coordination of policies of management, and the development there from of experimental research teams. Such organisation and statistical assessment of the results has been dominated now for decades by the work of Sir Herbert Seddon. It was in fact a whole decade after the war before he published the superlative summary *Peripheral Nerve Injuries* by the Nerve Injury Committee, London 1951.

Professor Merle d'Aubigné highlighted aspects of progress during the 1950s and 1960s: in specialisation of surgical facilities; in physiology; in clinical investigation, particularly electromyography; in surgical advances, in both technique and the use of the operating microscope. Post-operatively, greater understanding of physiological and clinical data had played a part in rehabilitation. But he made the point that the surgical understanding of nerve injuries had been dominated for decades by one man: Herbert Seddon.

The best surgeons of the twentieth century were regarded with awe by the public and even more so by their juniors. They became powerful autocrats who could endorse or ruin a young man's career (for surgery was almost exclusively a male profession). Even in the 1950s in the National Health Service, the consultant continued to wield tremendous power in 'his' hospital and imposed discipline on junior staff. Seddon built his career on hard work and the highest possible standards, as well as natural talent. He expected the same of those who worked for him, so being seen as an autocrat, role model and teacher was all part of the job. His public face contrasted with his private life: with his family and a wide circle of interesting friends and colleagues he showed a strong sense of humour and a boyish sense of fun. Despite a heavy work load, he made time for other activities, such as climbing, gardening and painting, and for attendance at church.

Mary often worried about Jim's health. Not only did he have 'poor digestion' but he had heart trouble too. Ill health prevented him from attending the BOA autumn meeting in Birmingham in 1973. In his final years he often needed oxygen, and cylinders were kept in the house. Over the years he had feared cancer of the gut and from time to time he would ask a reluctant colleague to palpate his abdomen for lumps or even to give a rectal examination. His final illness was abdominal; he went into hospital for surgery, from which he never recovered. He died on 21 December 1977. At the private funeral held at St John's Church, Stanmore, instead of flowers, donations were requested for the Organ Restoration Fund and for Christian Aid.

His life was celebrated on 27 January 1978 in a service of thanksgiving at St John's, attended by many friends, former colleagues and prominent figures from the medical and surgical worlds, and beyond, among them Sir John McMichael, Director of the British Postgraduate Medical Federation, Professor JIP James from Edinburgh, Lloyd Roberts representing the British Orthopaedic Association, Lord Briggs representing Worcester College, Oxford, an Air Marshal and senior officers from the RAF, the Mayor and Mayoress of Harrow, and governors from his old school at Hulme, Manchester, to name but a few.[173]

The Rector of St John's, the Revd Michael Bowles, gave the address and described Jim Seddon as a ten-talent man, a reference to the sermon Seddon had recently given on the parable of the talents. In that sermon he had shared his own philosophy of life with the congregation: "he believed that all of us have received from God talents and he believed that one day we shall be required to give an account of how we have used them. And as he believed, so he lived." A service of thanksgiving was also held by the Royal National Orthopaedic Hospital and the Institute of Orthopaedics on 17 February, when Donal Brooks gave the address and lightened the occasion with the story of Seddon's operation on an unwilling donkey (see p. 83-84).

36.
Cremation plaque

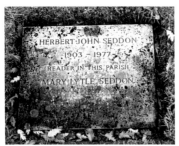

A cremation plaque (no. J159 in the List of Memorials by Humphrey Ward, 2004) was placed in the churchyard of St John the Evangelist Church, Stanmore, in memory of him and later of his wife, who missed him severely. The white lead lettering simply reads:

Herbert John Seddon
1903–1977
Reader in this Parish
Mary Lytle Seddon 1903–1983

173 *Harrow Observer* (Friday 3 February 1978), p. 2.

Robert Merle d'Aubigné wrote:

il avait gardé une merveilleuse simplicité. La figure …
un peu sévère était presque toujours égayée d'un sourire
parfois ironique, même sarcastique, mais dominé par la
bienveillance. Ses interventions et ses remarques,
publiques ou privées, toujours objectifes et aux termes
soigneusement pesés étaient, bien souvent, entrecoupés
par une incidente humoristique: il savaient être sérieux
et léger à la fois.[174]

His importance to the RNOH was appropriately marked
when the physiotherapy department was converted into a postgraduate teaching centre in 1984 and named the Sir Herbert Seddon
Centre. His portrait hangs in the entrance, and photographs of many
of the great names in orthopaedics hang along the corridor. In 1991
Seddon was further honoured when Professor Bentley, head of the
RNOH at the time, founded the Seddon Society. The inaugural meeting in June ended with a dinner and dance to the music of The
Vintage Hot Orchestra. The Seddon Society's first aim is: "To pro-
mote fellowship and professional links between surgeons who have
received a significant proportion of their orthopaedic training at the
Royal National Orthopaedic Hospital Trust". A further aim is to pro-
mote the RNOH and Institute of Orthopaedics as the "foremost"
orthopaedic centre in Great Britain. The society's badge is the tree of
André, with SS twined round the crooked trunk (representing defor-
mity) and the straight staff (representing orthopaedic treatment). It
was just 250 years since André had defined *orthopaedia* as the art of
preventing and correcting deformities in children.

The last words must be about his professional career. Alan
Lettin summed up the all-round gifts and dedication of his old chief:
"Jim was a good anatomist and a good operator, he knew how to
direct research and he was a good clinician". To which we may add
this from a patient who had arrived at the hospital paralysed and

---

'174 He retained a wonderful simplicity. His expression … which was a
little severe was nearly always brightened with a smile, sometimes iron-
ic, even sarcastic, but dominated by kindness. His speeches and comments, public or private, always objective and in terms carefully
weighed, were quite often interspersed with something humorous: he
knew how to be both serious and light at the same time.'

despondent: "His understanding and courtesy as well as a friendly and civilised atmosphere of the whole hospital (produced I am sure by his example and influence) gave me new hope".

His book, *Surgical Disorders of the Peripheral Nerves*, lives on. In 1998 it was revised by Rolfe Birch (consultant at the RNOH and, among other posts, orthopaedic surgeon to the Royal Navy), George Bonney (St Mary's) and CB Wynn Parry (former Director of Rehabilitation at RNOH) and now, at the time of writing seventy years after Seddon's arrival in Oxford, it is being revised again by Rolfe Birch. Professor Birch warns against the refusal to consider the physiological consequences of nerve injuries by using recent anatomical classifications. This is his opinion:

It is no more than a matter of historical fact that the work of Seddon and his colleagues, and he was fortunate in them, stands out as one of the most successful collaborations between alert and dedicated clinical and laboratory scientists. That work underpins most of what passes for 'modern' treatment of nerve injuries. I believe that the three most important and the most lasting contributions are as follows:

1. The analysis of the response to nerve injury,
2. The analysis of repair of gaps by nerve graft or by other methods,
3. Meticulous clinical examination, careful recording of clinical evidence, the scrupulous analysis of data which is collected prospectively as far as possible, and measurement of outcome.

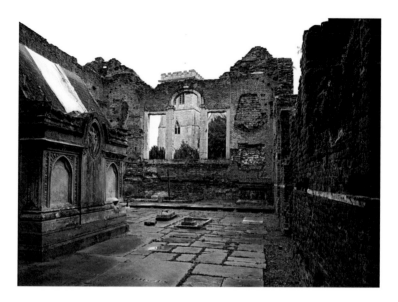

37. The St John's Church, Stanmore and the old church

Appendix

<u>Nerve Injuries Committee of the Medical Research Council [1954]</u>

HJ Seddon, CMG, DM, FRCS (Chairman)
EA Carmichael, CBE, MB, FRCP
Professor WE Le Gros Clark, MD, Dsc, FRCS, FRS
M Critchley, MD, FRCP
JG Greenfield, MD Bsc, FRCP
Professor Sir Geoffrey Jefferson, CBE, MS, FRCS, FRCP, FRS
Professor Sir James Learmonth, KCVO, CBE, ChM, FRCSE
Professor Sir Harry Platt, MD, MS, FRCS
Sir Charles Symonds, KBE, CB, DM, FRCP
Professor JZ Young, MA, FRS
FJC Herrald, MB, MRCPE (secretary).

References

BJS   *British Journal of Surgery*
BMJ   *British Medical Journal*
JBJS   *British Journal of Bone and Joint Surgery*
JRIPHH *Journal of the Royal Institute of Public Health and Hygiene*
PRSM *Proceedings of the Royal Society of Medicine*

Seddon's publications
The publications of Sir Herbert Seddon in chronological order

As sole author
1930 'Haemophilia as a cause of lesions in the nervous system', *Brain*, **53**, 306

1932a 'Calcaneo-scaphoid coalition', *PRSM*, **26** 419–424

1932b 'Volkmann's contracture', Letter. *BMJ*, **2**, No. 3734 (July 1932), 223

1934 'Pott's paraplegia', *BJS*, **22** (1934–5) p769

1935a 'Pott's paraplegia: prognosis and treatment', *BJS*, Vol. 22, No. 88 (April 1935)

1935b 'The morbid anatomy of caries of the thoracic spine in relation to treatment', *Lancet* (17 August 1935), 355–361

1936a 'Arthrodesis for tuberculosis of the hip in children', *St Bartholomew's Hospital Report*, **69** 199

1936b 'Treatment of spondylolisthesis', Letters. *BMJ*, **2**, No. 3956 (October 1936), 894, and No. 3959 (November 1936), 1053

1937 'Necrosis head of femur following fracture in a child', *PRSM*, **30** (1936-7) i, 210

1938a 'Treatment of tuberculous disease of the spine in adults', *PRSM*, **31** 951–958

1938b 'Angle of abduction of the hip after sub-trochanteric osteotomy', *Lancet*, Vol. 232, No. 6001 (3 September 1938), 549–602 II 552

1939 'Inguinal lymph gland biopsy in the diagnosis of tuberculous disease of the knee', *BMJ*, **1**, No. 4072 (21 January 1939), 105–107

1940 'Treatment of irrecoverable paralysis after poliomyelitis', *BMJ*, **1**, No. 4125 (January 1940), 139–141, and No. 4126 (February 1940), 182–185

1942a 'A classification of nerve injuries', *BMJ*, **2**, No. 4260 (29 August 1942), 237–239

1942b 'Injuries of the peripheral nerves', in Bailey H, *Surgery of Modern Warfare*, 2nd edn, Vol. 2, pp. 551–577, Edinburgh: E & S Livingstone [also revised version as Chapter 59 in Vol. 2 of 3rd edn, 1944]

1943a 'Three types of nerve Injury', *Brain*, **66**, part 4, 237–288

1943b 'Peripheral nerves' [special contribution], *British Medical Bulletin*, 1, No. 7

1943c 'Peripheral nerve injuries', *Glasgow Medical Journal*, **139** (March 1943), 61–75

1943d 'Peripheral nerve injuries' in H Bailey, *Surgery of modern warfare*, 3rd edn, E & S Livingstone, Edinburgh and London, Vol. 2, p. 551

1944 'The early management of peripheral nerve injuries', *Practitioner*, **152**, 101

1945a 'A short history of scrofula' [paper read on 17 January at the Royal University, Malta British Medical Journal, Malta Branch], Criterion Press, Valletta, Malta.

1945b 'The private citizen and the public heath' *Proceedings of the Royal Society of Arts and Sciences of Mauritius*, 1945

1945c 'The treatment of lower motor neuron lesions,1945' *Journal of the Chartered Society of Physiotherapy*, lecture to the congress 29 September 1944

1946a 'The pathology of Pott's paraplegia', *PRSM*, **29** 723

1946b 'Discussion on spinal caries with paraplegia', *PRSM*, **39** 723–734

1946c Seddon HJ, Hawes EIB and Raffray JR, 'The poliomyelitis epidemic in Mauritius in 1945', *Lancet*, Vol. 248, No. 6429 (16 November 1946), 703–738 [2 207]

1947a 'Nerve lesions complicating certain closed bone injuries', *Journal of the American Medical Association*, **135**, 691–694

1947b 'The use of autogenous grafts for the repair of large gaps in peripheral nerves', *BJS*, **35**, No. 138 (October 1947), 151–167

1947c 'The use of autogenous grafts for the repair of large gaps in peripheral nerves' [Charles Mayo Lecture], *Quarterly Bulletin of Northwestern University Medical School*, **21**, 201

1947d 'The early treatment of poliomyelitis', *BMJ*, **2**, No. 4521 (August 1947), 319–321

1947e 'Infantile paralysis', *JRIPHH*, **10** 382

1947f 'The practical value of peripheral nerve repair', *PRSM*, **42** 427

1948a 'The after treatment of poliomyelitis', *Practitioner*, **160** 195

1948b 'War injuries of peripheral nerves', *BJS* Suppl. 2, 325–353
1948c 'Brachial plexus' in *British Surgical Practice*, ed. ER Carling and JP Ross, London: Butterworth
1948d 'Comment re Ramshoff', *JBJS*, **30B**, 386
1949 'Brachial plexus injuries', *JBJS*, **31B** (February 1949), 3–4
1952 'Carpal ganglion as a cause of paralysis of the deep branch of the ulnar nerve', *JBJS*, **34B** (August 1952), 386–390
1953 'Poliomyelitis' [book review] *JBJS* **35B** (August 1953), p.510
1954 *Peripheral Nerve Injuries*, Medical Research Council Report Series No. 282, ed. HJ Seddon. London: Her Majesty's Stationery Office
1956 'Volkmann's contracture. Treatment by excision of the infarct', *JBJS*, **38B** (February 1956), 152–174
1957a 'Chirurgie orthopédique des paralysies', ed. R Merle d'Aubigné [book review], *JBJS*, **39B**, 602–603
1957b 'Knock-knee in children' [correspondence], *BMJ*, **2**: 1303
1957c 'Outline of Fractures, including Joint Injuries' [Book review] *BMJ*, **2**: 396
1959 'A dilettante view of surgery in East Africa', *East Africa Medical Journal*, **36**: 350.
1961a 'The scientific surgeon' [presidential address: BOA, Manchester, 14 April 1961], *JBJS*, **43B** (November 1961), 628–633
1961b 'The Manchester Ship Canal and the Colonial Frontier' [Robert Jones Lecture: RCS Eng., 8 Decem 1960], *JBJS*, **43B** (August 1961) 3, 425–43
1962a 'Dislocation of the hip' [editorial], *JBJS*, **44B** (May 1962), 255–256
1962b *Fitness Medicine*, London: Tyndale Press for the Christian Medical Fellowship.
1963 'Nerve grafting' [The 4th Watson-Jones Lecture], *JBJS*, **45B** (August 1963), 447–461
1964 'Volkmann's ischaemia' [The 4th Ruscoe Clarke Memorial Lecture], *BMJ*, **1**, 1587–1592
1966a 'Orthopaedic surgery', *BJS*, Vol. 53, No. 10 (October 1966) 836–839
1966b 'Volkmann's ischaemia in the lower limb', *JBJS*, **48B** (November 1966), 627–636
1967 'Nerve suture and nerve grafts in the upper limb', *10ème Congres de la Société Internationale de Chirurgie Orthopédique et de Traumatologie*, Brussels: Acta Medica Belgica, p. 739
1969 'Nerves and Nerve Injuries' [book review], *JBJS*, **51**, 583

1970 'Great teachers of surgery in the past', *JBJS* **52B**, 197
1972 *Surgical Disorders of the Peripheral Nerves*, 1st edn, Edinburgh and London: Churchill Livingstone.
1972a 'Peripheral Nerve Lesions' [book review], *BMJ* Vol. 3, No. 5822 (August 1972), 359
1974 *New Developments on myography and clinical neurophysiology.* Ed John E. Desmedt [book review]. *JBJS*
1975 *Surgical Disorders of the Peripheral Nerves*, 2nd edn, Edinburgh and London: Churchill Livingstone.
1976 'The choice of treatment in Pott's disease', *JBJS*, **58B** (November 1976), 395–397
1977 'In memoriam: Joseph Trueta', *JBJS* (1977) **59**, 243

As joint author

1926 Alexander GL and Seddon HJ, 'A case of cervical dislocation and paraplegia with recovery', *BJS*, Vol. 14 , No. 54 (October 1926) 365–637
1937 Fitzgerald FP and Seddon HJ, 'Lambrinudi's operation for drop foot', *BJS*, Vol. 25, No. 98 (October 1937), pp. 283–292
1940 Seddon HJ and St Clair Strange FG, 'Sacro-iliac tuberculosis', *BJS*, Vol. 28, No. 110 (October 1940) 193–221
1942 Seddon HJ and Medawar PB, 'Fibrin suture of human nerves', *Lancet*, **2**, 87
1942 Seddon HJ, Young JZ and Holmes W, 'The histological condition of a nerve autograft in man', *BJS*, **29**, No. 116 (April 1942), 378
1942 Seddon HJ and Florey HW, 'Filter cloth for controlling smell from plasters', *Lancet*, **1**, 755
1943 Seddon HJ, Medawar PB and Smith HV, 'Rate of regeneration of peripheral nerves in man', *Journal of Physiology* [London], **102**, 191
1944 Seddon HJ and Holmes W, 'Late condition of nerve homografts in man', *Surgery, Gynecology & Obstetrics*, **79**, 342
1944 Holmes W, Highet WB and Seddon HJ, 'Ischaemic nerve lesions occurring in Volkmann's contracture', *BJS*, Vol. 32, No. 126 (October 1944) 259–275
1945 Seddon HJ and Holmes W, 'Ischaemic damage in the peripheral stump of a divided nerve', *BJS*, **32**, No. 127 (January 1945), 389–391
1945 Seddon HJ, Agius T, Bernstein HGG and Tunbridge RE, *The Poliomyelitis Epidemic in Malta*, 1942–43 (received 28 August

1944, this was an offprint from the *JRIPHH* and also published in Quarterly Journal of Medicine, Vol. 14, No. 1 (January 1945), 1–26 [**38**: 1–26]

1945 Agius T, Bartolo AE, Coleiro C and Seddon HJ, 'Clinical features of the poliomyelitis epidemic in Malta, 1942–43', *BMJ*, **1**, No. 4404 (June 1945), 759–763

1945 Jackson ECS and Seddon HJ, 'Influence of galvanic stimulation on muscle atrophy resulting from denervation', *BMJ*, **2**, No. 4423 (October 1945), 485–486 and 622.

1946 McFarlan AM, Dick GWA and Seddon HJ, 'The epidemiology of the 1945 outbreak of poliomyelitis in Mauritius', *Quarterly Journal of Medicine*, new series **15** (1946) 59, 183–208.

1946 Seddon HJ, Hawes EIB and Raffray JR, 'The poliomyelitis epidemic in Mauritius in 1945', *Lancet*, Vol. 248, No. 6429, 707–712

1949 Seddon HJ and Riddoch G, 'Surgery of peripheral nerves', *BJS* Suppl. 517–533

1953 Muller EM and Seddon HJ, 'Late results of treatment of congenital dislocation of the hip', *JBJS*, **35B** (August 1953) 3, 342–362

1953 Seddon HJ and Riddoch G, 'Surgery of the peripheral nerves', Chapter 11 in *Surgery*, ed. VZ Cope, London: HMSO, pp. 245–6.

1954 Seddon HJ (ed.), *Peripheral Nerve Injuries*, Medical Research Council Special Report Series No. 282

1956 Griffiths DLl, Seddon HJ and Roaf R, *Pott's Paraplegia*, Oxford: Oxford University Press

1957 Nicholson DR and Seddon HJ, 'Nerve repair in civil practice. Results of treatment of median and ulnar nerve lesions', *BMJ*, **2** (November 1957) 5053, 1065–1071

1959 Brooks DN and Seddon HJ, 'Pectoral transplantation for paralysis of flexors of elbow – a new technique', *JBJS*, **41B** (February 1959), 36–43

1959 Segal A, Seddon HJ and Brooks DM, 'Treatment of the flexors of the elbow', *JBJS*, **41B**, 44–50

1960 Clawson DK and Seddon HJ, 'The results of repair of the sciatic nerve' and 'Late consequences of sciatic nerve injury', *JBJS*, **42B** (May 1960) 2, 205–212 and 213–225

1960 Mackenzie IG, Seddon HJ and Trevor D, 'Congenital dislocation of the hip', *JBJS*, **42B** (November 1960), 689–705

1961 Yeoman PM and Seddon HJ, 'Brachial plexus injuries: treatment

of the flail arm', *JBJS*, **43B** (August 1961) 3, 493–500
1964 Seddon HJ and Kirkaldy-Willis WH, 'In memoriam: Clifford Viney Braimbridge', *JBJS*, **46B** (1964), 350–351
1965 Leffert RD and Seddon HJ, 'Infraclavicular brachial plexus injuries', *JBJS*, **47B** (February 1965), 9–22
1966 Howse AJG and Seddon HJ, 'Ischaemic contracture of muscle associated with carbon monoxide and barbiturate poisoning', *BMJ*, **585** (1966), 192–5
1968 Parsons DW and Seddon HJ, 'The results of operations for disorders of the hip caused by poliomyelitis', *JBJS*, **50B** (May 1968), 266–273
1971 Seddon HJ and Howse AJ, 'Bullous lesions in poisoning', Letter. *BMJ*, Vol. 3 No. 5770 (August 1971), 371

Other references

In alphabetical order
BJS   *British Journal of Surgery*
BMJ   *British Medical Journal*
BON   *British Orthopaedic News*
JBJS   *British Journal of Bone and Joint Surgery*

Abercrombie RG, 'Galvanic stimulation of denervated muscle' [correspondence], *BMJ* (1945) 622
Agius T, Bartolo AE, Coleiro C and Seddon HJ, 'Clinical features of the poliomyelitis epidemic in Malta, 1942–43', *BMJ*, **1**, No. 4404 (June 1945), 759–763
Alexander GL and Seddon HJ, 'A case of cervical dislocation and paraplegia with recovery', *BJS*, Vol. 14 , No. 54 (October 1926) 365–367
Aubigné M d', Preface in Vol. 2 of *Traumatic lesions of the upper limb*, ed. J Michon and E Moberg, trans. from French by E Moberg for GEM and the Committee on Nerve Injuries. Edinburgh and London: Churchill Livingstone
Bakker E, Reminiscences [of Leendert Jonker], WW2 People's War Article A1154341 (2004) [online] BBC website. URL http://www.rafcommands.com/cgi-bin/dcforum/dcboard.cgi Forum: DCForumID6 Thread Number: 4403
Bernstein HGG, Clark TMP and Tunbridge RE, 'Acute anterior poliomyelitis among service personnel in Malta', *BMJ*, **1** (1945), 763–767

Birch R, Bonney G and Wynn Parry CB, *Surgical Disorders of the Peripheral Nerves*. London: Churchill Livingstone (1998).

Bonney G, 'The value of axon responses in determining the site of lesion in fraction injuries of the brachial plexus', *Brain*, **77** (1954), 588

Bonney GLW, 'Obituary: Donal Brooks', *Journal of Hand Surgery*, **30B** (2004), 97–98

Bowden REM, 'Changes in human voluntary muscle in denervation and re-inervation', *BMJ*, **2** (1945), 487–488

BOA Edinburgh meeting report. McQuilllan WM 'New isolation techniques as adjunct to secondary nerve repair' comment by Seddon on the use of millipore. *JBJS*, **49B** (1966) 186

Brain WR, 'Encounters with Winston Churchill', *Medical History*, **44** (2000), 1: 3–20

Brooks DN and Seddon HJ, 'Pectoral transplantation for paralysis of the flexors of the elbow – a new technique', *JBJS*, **41B** (February 1959), 36–43

Brooks DM, 'In memoriam Sir Herbert Seddon', *JBJS*, **60B** (1978) 2, 278

Carver M, *The Lord Harding of Petherton GLB, CBE, DSO, MC, 1896–1989*. London: Weidenfeld & Nicolson (1978)

Caughey JE and Porteous WM, *Medical Journal of Australia*, **1** (1946), 5–10

Cholmeley JA, *History of the Royal National Orthopaedic Hospital*. London: Chapman & Hall (1985)

Clarke O, 'Appreciation' [Harry Platt Birthday Volume], *JBJS*, **48B** (1966), 614

Clawson DK and Seddon HJ, 'The results of repair of the sciatic nerve' and 'Late consequences of sciatic nerve injury', *JBJS*, **42B** (1960) 2, 205–212 and 213–215

d'Aubigné *see* Aubigné

Davis L, Neurological Surgery Ch 4 p392—410 and p294 In: *Activities of Surgical Consultants*. Vol 2 The Medical Department United States Army in World War II, Washington DC(1964) Library of Congress Catalogue card no. 62-60004

Davis L, Peripheral Nerve Grafts. Ch. 20 Activities of Surgical Consultants. In: *Neurosurgery* vol 2 p493 The Medical Department United States Army in World War II, Washington (1958–9)

Editorial: 'Joint Meeting of the English-Speaking Orthopaedic Associations', *JBJS*, **34** (1952), 3–5.

Fitzgerald FP and Seddon HJ, 'Lambrinudi's operation for drop foot',

BJS, Vol. **25**, No. 98 (October 1937), pp. 283–292

Fletcher C, 'First clinical trial of penicillin', *BMJ*, **289** (1984), 1721

Galea J, Introduction in *Melita Historica, Journal of the Malta Historical Society* (1952), 33–49

Griffiths DLl, Seddon HJ and Roaf R, *Pott's Paraplegia*, Oxford: Oxford University Press

Guttmann L, 'Topographical studies of disturbances of sweat secretion after complete lesions of the peripheral nerves', *Journal of Neurology, Neurosurgery and Psychiatry*, **3** (1940), 197

Harrison M [2004a] *Medicine and Victory: British Medical History in the Second World War*, Oxford: Oxford University Press (2004), p. 54 [reference 66 to Imperial War Museum 87/9/1(P), Diaries of Miss EM Luker; Queen Alexandra Imperial Nursing Service, Diary of 1940 No. 12 Casualty Clearing Station, France]

Harrison M [2004b] Public Records Office, War Office 222/120, 'Report on surgery in the Dieppe Raid 3' in Harrison, *Medicine and Victory*, Oxford: Oxford University Press (2004), 237–8

Highet E, Reminiscences WW2 People's War, articles AD4047509 and AD4047978 (2005) [online]
http://www.bbc.co.uk/ww2peopleswar/stories/09/a4047509shtml
http://www.bbc.co.uk/ww2peopleswar/stories/78/a4047978shtml

Highet WB and Holmes W, 'Traction injuries to the peripheral nerves after surgery', *BJS*, **30** (1943), 212

Highet WB, Bremner and Sanders FK, 'Effect of stretching nerves after suture', *BJS*, **30** (1943), 355–371

Holmes W, Highet WB and Seddon HJ, 'Ischaemic nerve lesions occurring in Volkmann's contracture', *BJS*, Vol. 32, No. 126 (October 1944) 259–275

Howse AJG and Seddon HJ, 'Ischaemic contracture of muscle associated with carbon monoxide and barbiturate poisoning', *BMJ*, **585** (1966), 192–5

Hulbert K, 'An echo of the past: the day war broke out', *BON*, Winter (1990–91), No.3, p.7

Jackson ECS and Seddon HJ, 'Influence of galvanic stimulation on muscle atrophy resulting from denervation', *BMJ*, **2**, No. 4423 (October 1945), 485–486 and 622

James JIP, 'In memoriam: Herbert Seddon', *JBJS*, **60B** (1978) 2, 276-277

Jellinek EH, 'Sir Harold Stiles (1863–1946)', *Journal of Medical Biography*, **6** (1998), 128–133

Kemp H, 'John Cholmeley: 90th birthday', *BON*, Spring (1993), No.7, p.8

Kirkaldy-Willis WH and Wood AM (eds), *Principles of the Treatment of Trauma, Basic Principles, Plastic and Orthopaedic Aspects of Trauma*, with forewords by WR Mowlem and HJ Seddon. Edinburgh and London: E. & S. Livingstone (1962)

Kocher T, *Textbook of Operative Surgery*, 3rd English edn, trans. from 5th German edn by HJ Stiles and PC Balfour. London: A & C Black (1911)

Leffert RD and Seddon HJ, 'Infraclavicular brachial plexus injuries', *JBJS*, **47B** (February 1965), 9–22

Mackenzie IG, Seddon HJ and Trevor D, 'Congenital dislocation of the hip', *JBJS*, **42B** (November 1960), 689–705

McFarlan AM, Dick GWA and Seddon HJ, 'The epidemiology of the 1945 outbreak of poliomyelitis in Mauritius', *Quarterly Journal of Medicine*, new series **15** (1946) 59, 183–208

Milsom C, 'The first half-century of orthopaedic surgery in New Zealand', *JBJS*, **32B** (1950) 4, pp. 611–614 at 612.

The Medical Department United States Army in World War II, Washington. 1958 & 9.
Ch 1 The European Theatre of Operations p.71, Ch 20 Peripheral Nerve Grafts p493 *Neurosurgery* vol 2 Surgery in World War II Office of the Surgeon General Department of the Army. (see also Davis L, Spurling R Glen)

Moran, Lord, *Winston Churchill: The Struggle for Survival, 1940–1965*. London: Constable (1966)

Morley AJM, 'Knock-knee in children', *BMJ*, **2** (1957), 976–9 October.

Muller GM and Seddon HJ, 'Late results of treatment of congenital dislocation of the hip', *JBJS*, **35B** (August 1953) 3, 342–362.

Nicholson DR and Seddon HJ, 'Nerve repair in civil practice. Results of treatment of median and ulnar nerve lesions', *BMJ*, **2** (November 1957) 5053, 1065–1071.

Parsons DW and Seddon HJ, 'The results of operations for disorders of the hip caused by poliomyelitis', *JBJS* **50B** (May 1968), 266–273.

Paul JR, *History of Poliomyelitis*. New Haven CT and London: Yale University Press (1971)

Platt H and Bristow R, *Report to the International Society of Surgeons* (1923)

Pott P, *The Chirurgical Works of Percival Pott*, Vol. 3, London : printed for T. Lowndes, J. Johnson, G. Robinson, T. Cadell, T. Evans, W. Fox, J. Bew, and S. Hayes, (1779) Reminiscences of the

Wingfield Morris Hospital. Centre for Oxfordshire
Rocyn Jones A, 'A review of orthopaedic surgery in Britain', *JBJS*, **38B**
(February 1956) 1
Royal Society of Medicine Archives, Section on Orthopaedics. Council
records
Scales JT, 'The use of polythene and resinated asbestos felt for splints',
JBJS, **32B** (1950), 60–65.
Segal A, Seddon HJ and Brooks DM, 'Treatment of the flexors of the
elbow', *JBJS*, **41B** (1959), 44–50
Shott GD, 'Nan West's murals in the National Orthopaedic Hospital',
BMJ, **317** (1998), No. 7174: 1736
S WS, 'Carl E Badgley', *JBJS*, **55A** (1973) 5, 1112–13
Spurling R Glen, Ch: *The European Theatre of Operation*. P71.Vol:
Neurosurgery. Surgery in World War ll. The Medical Department
United States Army in World War II, Washington DC (1958)
Stiles HJ and Forrester Brown MF, *Treatment of Injuries of Peripheral
Nerves*, Oxford Medical Publications. London: Henry Frowde
and Hodder & Stoughton (1922)
Stoker D, *BON*, No.12 (1995), p.34
Stuart D, 'The development of orthopaedics in Kenya – personal reflec-
tions', *BON*, No. 26 (2002), p.5
Trueta J, *Treatment of War Wounds and Fractures, with special refer-
ence to the closed method as used in the war in Spain*. London:
Hamish Hamilton (1939)
Trueta J, *The Principles and Practice of War Surgery, with special refer-
ence to the biological method of treatment of wounds and frac-
tures*. London: William Heinemann Medical (1943)
Trueta J, *The Spirit of Catalonia*. London (1946)
Trueta J, *Surgeon in War and Peace* [memoirs], trans. from Catalan by
Meli and Michael Strubel. London: Victor Gollancz (1980)
University of Oxford Archives, UR6/MD/13/8 (files 1–2), Medical
School: Nuffield Professorship of Orthopaedics 1937–49 and
other bodies, UR6/MD/13/8A Wingfield-Morris relations with
the University
University of Oxford Archives, FA6/13/1–4 Annual report for Nuffield
Committee for the Advancement of Medicine 1942-50
University of Oxford Archives, UR6/CQ/11/8A/2 Payment of staff for
work in Oxford. Profeesor Seddon trips to Malta and Mauritius
Van Rooyen CE and Morgan AD, 'Poliomyelitis: experimental work in
Egypt', *Edinburgh Medical Journal*, **50** (1943), 705–720
Watson-Jones R, Preface in *Fractures and Joint Injuries*, 3rd edn.

Edinburgh and London: E & S Livingstone (1943)

Waugh W, *A History of the British Orthopaedic Association*. London: BOA (1993)

Weddell G, Feinstein B and Pattle RE, 'The clinical application of electromyography', *Lancet*, **1** (1943), 236–239 and Brain 67 (1944), 178–257

Wingfield-Morris Orthopaedic Hospital Annual Reports 1944–1948

Yeoman PM and Seddon HJ, 'Brachial plexus injuries: treatment of the flail arm', *JBJS*, **43B** (August 1961) 3, 493–500

Young JZ, 'The functional repair of nervous tissue', *Physiological Reviews*, **22** (1942), 318

Young JZ, Introduction in *Peripheral Neuropathy*, ed. PJ Dyck. Philadelphia and London: WB Saunders (1993), pp. 2–5

Zachary RB and Roaf R, Chapter 3 in *Peripheral Nerve Injuries*, ed. HJ Seddon, Medical Research Council Special Report Series No. 282. London: HMSO (1954), 57–58

Index of Names